SO-ESD-888

NURSING DIAGNOSIS MANUAL for the Well and Ill Client

C. AUDEAN DUESPOHL, R.N., M.S.N., M.Ed.

Dean, School of Nursing
Clarion University of Pennsylvania,
Oil City, Pennsylvania

1986

W. B. SAUNDERS COMPANY

*Philadelphia, London, Toronto, Mexico City
Rio de Janeiro, Sydney, Tokyo, Hong Kong*

W. B. Saunders Company: West Washington Square
                          Philadelphia, PA 19105

Library of Congress Cataloging-in-Publication Data

Duespohl, T. Audean.
    Nursing diagnosis manual for the well and ill client.
    1. Diagnosis. 2. Nursing. I. Title. [DNLM:
1. Nursing Process. WY 100 D832n]
RT48.D84 1986   610.73   85-27661
ISBN 0-7216-1825-1

Editor: Dudley Kay

Developmental Editor: Alan Sorkowitz

Designer: Lorraine B. Kilmer

Production Manager: Frank Polizzano

Manuscript Editor: Edna Dick

Nursing Diagnosis Manual for the Well and Ill Client

                                        ISBN 0-7216-1825-1

Last digit is the print number: 9 8 7 6 5 4 3 2 1

To my sister and best friend, Bev Renninger
....who says, "It's about time!"

ACKNOWLEDGMENTS

My deepest appreciation is extended to my colleague and friend, Mary Kavoosi, whose honest advice and editorial support made an idea materialize into this manual.

My gratitude is offered to Dudley R. Kay, Publisher, Nursing and Allied Health, from W.B. Saunders Company who encouraged the publication of this manual.

My very special thanks goes to my family:

- My husband Terry, whose patience, understanding, and support makes anything possible.

- My daughter from Turkey, Fulay Cihan, who unselfishly shared her "Mom" during her year in the United States.

T.A.D.

CONTENTS

INTRODUCTION TO THE MANUAL

Nursing, as a practice discipline, is an emerging profession. It is seeking to be recognized as a profession through the promotion of the nursing process as the conceptual framework for nursing practice. Nursing diagnosis, as a vital component of the nursing process, describes the essence of the practice of professional nursing.

Just as the nursing process provides a basis for nursing practice, nursing diagnosis gives direction for activities of therapeutic nursing intervention. Moritz stressed the importance of nursing diagnosis to nursing when she defined it as a label for a client condition (response to health or illness) that professional nurses are able and legally responsible to treat (Moritz, 1982).

The act of diagnosing has long been accepted as a medical skill based on the pathological conditions of clients. The term *diagnosis* must now be shared by physicians with nursing since most nurse practice legislation in the United States identifies this process as a legal responsibility of the professional nurse. The New York State Nurse Practice Act is an example of an up-to-date legislative document that states:

> The practice of the profession of nursing as a registered professional nurse is defined as diagnosing and treating human responses to actual or potential health problems through such services as case finding, health teaching, health counseling, and provision of care supportive to or restorative of life and well-being....

The challenge to the professional nurse is to accept this

legal responsibility and provide quality nursing care through the use of nursing diagnosis.

THE CHALLENGE

Nursing diagnosis is the future for professional nursing and is acknowledged as such by nurse educators, administrators, and practitioners. However, lack of consistency in the use of nursing diagnosis by members of the nursing profession presents a major problem. In many instances, nurses have used medical terminology such as hypertension, diabetes, surgery, barium enema, and postpartum as nursing diagnoses. Thus, the focus of nursing therapy has been on medical problems, pathological conditions, disease processes, and complications rather than human responses treatable by the professional nurse. Nursing professionals have recognized the problems created by this interpretation and have taken steps to standardize nursing diagnoses emphasizing nursing interventions rather than medically oriented activities.

The North American Nursing Diagnosis Association (NANDA, formerly known as the National Group for the Classification of Nursing Diagnosis) has published an approved list of nursing diagnostic categories that were accepted for clinical testing. This action provides a basis for standardizing nursing research and clinical practice. There has been much discussion concerning the use of the diagnostic categories and their application to the "real world" of nursing.

Many renowned professional nurses believe that any problem or response identified from assessment data, regardless of whether or not it corresponds to NANDA's approved list, can be called a nursing diagnosis as long as it is legally treatable by nurses. Others support the concept that all activities of professional nurses, whether medical or nursing oriented, can be categorized into nursing diagnoses. Many other nurses subscribe to neither philosophical framework but apply nursing diagnosis inconsistently to any given situation.

If standardization and common terminology are desired, nurses must refrain from "making up" nursing diagnoses. It would seem obvious that arbitrarily labeling health responses as nursing diagnoses would lead to confusion, misunderstanding, and thinking that is more appropriate for physicians. NANDA's list of categories can serve no purpose if it is not incorporated into the practice of professional nursing. Thus, members of the profession must promote and utilize NANDA's nursing diagnoses while judging their validity.

A mechanism has been developed, whereby individuals who find that the existing categories do not seem to match the needs they identify in the clinical setting, can submit new nursing diagnoses after research and testing. This procedure was developed by Marjorie Gordon in 1982 and provides a method of preparing diagnostic categories for consideration by NANDA. For further instructions on this, see *Guidelines for Preparing Diagnostic Categories* (Gordon, 1982).

THE MANUAL

Because of the profession's historical evolution, nursing tends to focus on health problems of ill clients rather than on health responses that can be exhibited by either well or ill clients. The medical model is still the basis of practice for many professional nurses. Therefore, it is understandable that existing material written about nursing diagnoses emphasizes ill clients and their health problems. Thus, a need was identified for a handbook of nursing diagnoses based on a nursing model that stressed all aspects of professional nursing practice. This manual relates wellness- and illness-oriented client responses and situations to the nursing diagnostic categories as identified by NANDA.

For the purpose of this text, *wellness* is defined as the condition of life in which one's human responses do not interfere with the activities of daily living. Within this context, individuals perceive themselves as being well, although their level of wellness may vary greatly. On the other hand, *illness* is defined as the state of being in which one is incapacitated to the extent that activities of daily living cannot be accomplished without assistance. Thus, individuals who are unable to function at their usual level view themselves as being ill whether it be physically or psychologically. This framework provides the basis of the material included in Sections I and II.

Section I is designed to provide a quick reference guide for identifying nursing diagnostic categories associated with certain client responses and situations. It indexes NANDA's nursing diagnostic categories according to related client responses and situations. Similar client responses and situations are clustered into groups under wellness and illness components in order to define clearly the separate areas of nursing practice. The wellness section is indexed under the following: (1) Developmental, (2) Emotional, (3) Environmental, (4) Maturational, (5) Physiological, and (6) Situational. Associated nursing diagnostic categories are alphabetized under each of the headings in the wellness-oriented part of this section. The illness portion includes seven categories: (1) General Illness, (2) Acute Care Setting, (3) Mental Health, (4) Mobility, (5) Nutrition, (6) Physical Health, and (7) Systems. The illness-oriented section is arranged identically to the wellness portion with the associated diagnostic categories listed alphabetically under each of the seven headings. For instructions on the use of Section I, see page 10.

Section II contains the list of diagnostic categories as approved by NANDA. Content under each diagnostic category includes the following five divisions:

Definition
In order to clarify the meaning of the diagnostic categories a definition of each is included as content. In those diagnostic categories that have definitions approved by NANDA the exact statement is used. For categories with no definitions, a definition was developed by the author to interpret the diagnostic category and maintain consistency. Those definitions not approved by NANDA but included for clarification are marked with the symbol †.

Defining Characteristics
The defining characteristics as approved by NANDA are listed under each diagnostic category. No additional characteristics were added and none were deleted. The critical defining characteristics as identified by NANDA are marked with the symbol (††)

Nursing Diagnoses Based on Identified Etiologies
According to accepted practice, nursing diagnosis and nursing diagnostic statement are synonymous. Therefore, in this manual, the term *nursing diagnosis* is used interchangeably with *nursing diagnostic statement*. A nursing diagnosis consists of two parts joined by "related to" and describes a client response and the associated influencing factors. The first part of statement describes an actual or potential condition of the client as identified through assessment data. This corresponds with the nursing diagnostic category as identified by NANDA. The second part of the statement reflects the influencing factors that contribute to the client response. The second part corresponds with the accepted etiologies for the diagnostic categories. In order for a nurs-

ing diagnosis to be complete it must contain:

- a diagnostic category
- the "related to" phrase
- an etiology

In order to eliminate confusion, the nursing diagnoses in each diagnostic category are identified according to the etiologies accepted by NANDA. That is, the etiologies are not listed separately, but instead are incorporated into the nursing diagnoses.

Wellness- and Illness-Oriented Groups

In most instances, each nursing diagnosis (diagnostic category and etiology) can apply to both well and ill clients. In order to emphasize this, the content under each nursing diagnosis is divided into wellness oriented and illness oriented portions.

Client Responses and/or Situations Needing Assessment

Under each of the headings, wellness and illness, there is an alphabetized list of related client responses and situations that should be assessed in order to make the identified nursing diagnosis. The client responses and situations that are included under the nursing diagnoses are not meant to be all-inclusive or exclusive, but instead are groups of responses and situations that can be used to begin the diagnosing process. The identification of additional data under each nursing diagnosis is expected as the nurse individualizes nursing care in the clinical setting.

The content in Section II provides a quick reference for review of the diagnostic categories and nursing diagnoses, as well as an organized listing of well and ill client responses and situations that can be associated with each. For instructions on the use of Section II, see page 101.

APPROVED NURSING DIAGNOSTIC CATEGORIES (NANDA)

Activity Intolerance
Activity Intolerance, Potential
Airway Clearance, Ineffective
Anxiety
Bowel Elimination, Alteration in: Constipation
Bowel Elimination, Alteration in: Diarrhea
Bowel Elimination, Alteration in: Incontinence
Breathing Pattern, Ineffective
Cardiac Output, Alteration in: Decreased
Comfort, Alteration in: Pain
Communication, Impaired Verbal
Coping, Family: Potential for Growth
Coping, Ineffective Family: Compromised
Coping, Ineffective Family: Disabling
Coping, Ineffective Individual
Diversional Activity Deficit
Family Process, Alteration in
Fear
Fluid Volume, Alteration in: Excess
Fluid Volume Deficit, Actual (1)
Fluid Volume Deficit, Actual (2)
Fluid Volume Deficit, Potential
Gas Exchange, Impaired
Grieving, Anticipatory
Grieving, Dysfunctional
Health Maintenance, Alteration in
Home Maintenance Management, Impaired
Injury, Potential for
Knowledge Deficit (Specify)
Mobility, Impaired Physical
Noncompliance (Specify)
Nutrition, Alteration in: Less Than Body Requirements
Nutrition, Alteration in: More Than Body Requirements

Nutrition, Alteration in: Potential for More Than Body Requirements

Oral Mucous Membrane, Alteration in

Parenting, Alteration in: Actual or Potential

Powerlessness

Rape Trauma Syndrome

Self-Care Deficit

Self-Concept, Disturbance in: Body Image, Self-Esteem, Role Performance, Personal Identity

Sensory-Perceptual Alteration: Visual, Auditory, Kinesthetic, Gustatory, Tactile, Olfactory

Sexual Dysfunction

Skin Integrity, Impairment of: Actual

Skin Integrity, Impairment of: Potential

Sleep Pattern Disturbance

Social Isolation

Spiritual Distress (Distress of the Human Spirit)

Thought Processes, Alteration in

Tissue Perfusion, Alteration in: Cerebral, Cardiopulmonary, Renal, Gastrointestinal, Peripheral

Urinary Elimination, Alteration in Patterns of

Violence, Potential for: Self-Directed or Directed at Others

REFERENCES

Gordon, M. *Guidelines for Nursing Diagnosis Development and Workshops*. In Kim, M. J. and Moritz, D. A. (Eds). *Classification of Nursing Diagnoses; Proceedings of the Third and Fourth National Conferences.* St. Louis: C.V. Mosby Co., 1982, pp. 339–345.

Moritz, D. A. *Nursing Diagnoses in Relation to the Nursing Process*. In Kim, M. J. and Moritz, D. A. (Eds). *Classification of Nursing Diagnoses; Proceedings of the Third and Fourth National Conferences*. St. Louis: C.V. Mosby Co., 1982, pp. 53–57.

State of Washington Nurse Practice Act, Title 18, Section 18, 88.050, 1973.

SECTION I

INDEX

Nursing Diagnostic Categories
According to
Client Responses
and
Situations

INTRODUCTION TO SECTION I

10

Section I indexes nursing diagnostic categories according to related client responses and situations. Client responses and situations are divided into wellness and illness components in order to define clearly the separate areas of nursing practice. The wellness section is indexed under the following: Developmental, Emotional, Environmental, Maturational, Physiological, and Situational. The section in the illness portion includes General Illness, Acute Care Setting, Mental Health, Mobility, Nutrition, Physical Health, and Systems.

This section is designed to provide a quick reference guide for identifying nursing diagnostic categories associated with certain client responses and situations. Since similar client responses and situations are clustered into groups under wellness and illness, the process for using this index can be described as follows:

1. Determine whether the response or the situation is wellness or illness oriented.
2. Select the appropriate section in which the response or situation would be classified.
3. Review the general groupings to locate the desired client response and/or situation.
4. Identify the diagnostic category that could be derived from the assessed client response and/or situation.
5. Evaluate the diagnostic categories for relevancy to the client response and/or situation.
6. Choose the most appropriate diagnostic category and review the corresponding nursing diagnoses in Section 2 of this manual.
7. Derive a nursing diagnosis from the identified diagnostic category.

WELLNESS ORIENTED CLIENT RESPONSES AND SITUATIONS

ILLNESS ORIENTED CLIENT RESPONSES AND SITUATIONS

14

WELLNESS ORIENTED

DEVELOPMENTAL

(This category is indexed chronologically instead of alphabetically in order to facilitate subject location.)

Birth

Infancy

Childhood

Adolescence

Young Adulthood

Middle Age

Agedness

EMOTIONAL

Abuse

Anorexia/Overeating

Anxiety

Coping

Depression

Emotions

Fear

Grieving

Habits

Noncompliance

Breathing Pattern, Ineffective, **136**
Coping, Ineffective Family: Disabling, **158**
Health Maintenance, Alteration in, **197**
Home Maintenance Management, Impaired, **203**
Knowledge Deficit, **217**
Parenting, Alteration in: Actual or Potential, **242**
Self-Care Deficit: Feeding, Bathing/Hygiene, Dressing/
   Grooming, Toileting, **256**

Powerlessness

Anxiety, **112**
Coping, Family: Potential for Growth, **151**
Coping, Ineffective Family: Compromised, **153**
Coping, Ineffective Family: Disabling, **158**
Coping, Ineffective Individual, **162**
Grieving, Anticipatory, **189**
Grieving, Dysfunctional, **191**
Health Maintenance, Alteration in, **197**
Parenting, Alteration in: Actual or Potential, **242**
Powerlessness, **252**
Sexual Dysfunction, **273**
Sleep Pattern Disturbance, **288**
Social Isolation, **292**

Rape Trauma

Anxiety, **112**
Coping, Ineffective Family: Disabling, **158**
Coping, Ineffective Individual, **162**
Family Process, Alteration in, **174**
Grieving, Anticipatory, **189**
Grieving, Dysfunctional, **191**
Injury, Potential for, **208**

Self-Concept

Social Isolation

Spiritual Distress

Stress/Distress

ENVIRONMENTAL

Altitude

Gas Exchange, Impaired, **186**
Self-Care Deficit: Feeding, Bathing/Hygiene, Dressing/
  Grooming, Toileting, **256**
Thought Processes, Alteration in, **301**
Tissue Perfusion, Alteration in: Cerebral, Cardiopulmon-
  ary, Renal, Gastrointestinal, Peripheral, **304**

Pollution

Anxiety, **112**
Bowel Elimination, Alteration in: Diarrhea, **128**
Injury, Potential for, **208**
Sensory-Perceptual Alteration: Visual, Auditory, Kines-
  thetic, Gustatory, Tactile, Olfactory, **269**

Sensory Deprivation Overload

Anxiety, **112**
Communication, Impaired Verbal, **148**
Fear, **176**
Health Maintenance, Alteration in, **197**
Home Maintenance Management, Impaired, **203**
Noncompliance, **226**
Nutrition, Alteration: More Than Body Requirements, **231**
Sensory-Perceptual Alteration: Visual, Auditory, Kines-
  thetic, Gustatory, Tactile, Olfactory, **269**
Social Isolation, **292**

Weather

Airway Clearance, Ineffective, **108**
Fear, **176**
Injury, Potential for, **208**
Skin Integrity, Impairment of: Actual, **279**
Skin Integrity, Impairment of: Potential, **287**
Sleep Pattern Disturbance, **288**

MATURATIONAL

Communication

Communication, Impaired Verbal, **148**
Coping, Family: Potential for Growth, **151**
Fear, **176**
Knowledge Deficit, **217**
Noncompliance, **226**
Nutrition, Alteration in: Less Than Body Requirements, **227**
Nutrition, Alteration in: More Than Body Requirements, **231**
Powerlessness, **252**
Self-Care Deficit: Feeding, Bathing/Hygiene, Dressing/Grooming, Toileting, **256**
Sensory-Perceptual Alteration: Visual, Auditory, Kinesthetic, Gustatory, Tactile, Olfactory, **269**
Thought Processes, Alteration in, **301**

Culture/Values

Anxiety, **112**
Coping, Ineffective Individual, **162**
Family Process, Alteration in, **174**
Fear, **176**
Nutrition, Alteration in: More Than Body Requirements, **231**
Nutrition, Alteration in: Potential for More Than Body Requirements, **233**
Powerlessness, **252**
Self-Concept, Disturbance in: Body Image, Self-Esteem, Role Performance, Personal Identity, **263**
Sexual Dysfunction, **273**
Social Isolation, **292**

32

Death

Anxiety, **112**
Coping, Family: Potential for Growth, **151**
Coping, Ineffective Family: Compromised, **153**
Coping, Ineffective Family: Disabling, **158**
Coping, Ineffective Individual, **162**
Grieving, Anticipatory, **189**
Grieving, Dysfunctional, **191**
Home Maintenance Management, Impaired, **203**
Parenting, Alteration in: Actual or Potential, **242**
Spiritual Distress, **298**

Family

Anxiety, **112**
Bowel Elimination, Alteration in: Constipation, **120**
Comfort, Alteration in: Pain, **144**
Coping, Family: Potential for Growth, **151**
Coping, Ineffective Family: Compromised, **153**
Coping, Ineffective Family: Disabling, **158**
Coping, Ineffective Individual, **162**
Family Process, Alteration in, **174**
Fear, **176**
Grieving, Anticipatory, **189**
Grieving, Dysfunctional, **191**
Home Maintenance Management, Impaired, **203**
Parenting, Alteration in: Actual or Potential, **242**
Self-Care Deficit: Feeding, Bathing/Hygiene, Dressing/
    Grooming, Toileting, **256**
Self-Concept, Disturbance in: Body Image, Self-Esteem,
    Role Performance, Personal Identity, **263**
Sensory-Perceptual Alteration: Visual, Auditory, Kines-
    thetic, Gustatory, Tactile, Olfactory, **269**
Sexual Dysfunction, **273**

Knowledge

34 Language

Parenting

Pregnancy

PHYSIOLOGICAL

Abortion

Allergies

Aspiration

Breathing

Circulatory Responses

Cough

Dental Problems/Protheses

Elimination

Exercise

Fatigue

Coping, Ineffective Individual, **162**
Injury, Potential for, **208**
Mobility, Impaired Physical, **221**
Self-Care Deficit: Feeding, Bathing/Hygiene, Dressing/
  Grooming, Toileting, **256**
Skin Integrity, Impairment of: Actual, **279**
Skin Integrity, Impairment of: Potential, **287**

Headache

Comfort, Alteration in: Pain, **144**
Mobility, Impaired Physical, **221**
Self-Care Deficit: Feeding, Bathing/Hygiene, Dressing/
  Grooming, Toileting, **256**

Infertility

Anxiety, **112**
Comfort, Alteration in: Pain, **144**
Coping, Family: Potential for Growth, **151**
Coping, Ineffective Family: Compromised, **153**
Coping, Ineffective Family: Disabling, **158**
Coping, Ineffective Individual, **162**
Family Process, Alteration in, **174**
Grieving, Anticipatory, **189**
Health Maintenance, Alteration in, **197**
Parenting, Alteration in: Actual or Potential, **242**
Self-Concept, Disturbance in: Body Image, Self-Esteem,
  Role Performance, Personal Identity, **263**
Sexual Dysfunction, **273**

Medications

Bowel Elimination, Alteration in: Diarrhea, **128**
Fluid Volume Deficit, Potential, **185**
Injury, Potential for, **208**

Mental Retardation

Mobility

Nutrition

Poisons

Coping, Ineffective Individual, **162**
Grieving, Anticipatory, **189**
Grieving, Dysfunctional, **191**
Health Maintenance, Alteration in, **197**
Nutrition, Alteration in: Less Than Body Requirements, **227**
Parenting, Alteration in: Actual or Potential, **242**
Powerlessness, **252**
Self-Care Deficit: Feeding, Bathing/Hygiene, Dressing/ Grooming, Toileting, **256**
Self-Concept, Disturbance in: Body Image, Self-Esteem, Role Performance, Personal Identity, **263**
Sexual Dysfunction, **273**
Sleep Pattern Disturbance, **288**
Social Isolation, **292**
Spiritual Distress, **298**
Thought Processes, Alteration in, **301**
Violence, Potential for: Self-Directed or Directed at Others, **311**

Weight/Height

Activity Intolerance, **104**
Anxiety, **112**
Bowel Elimination, Alteration in: Constipation, **120**
Breathing Pattern, Ineffective, **136**
Comfort, Alteration in: Pain, **144**
Coping, Family: Potential for Growth, **151**
Coping, Ineffective Family: Compromised, **153**
Coping, Ineffective Family: Disabling, **158**
Coping, Ineffective Individual, **162**
Fear, **176**
Fluid Volume Deficit, Potential, **185**
Grieving, Anticipatory, **189**
Grieving, Dysfunctional, **191**
Mobility, Impaired Physical, **221**

SITUATIONAL

Accidents

Crisis

Diagnostic Studies

Economic

Education

Employment

Incarceration

50

Life Style

Loss

Marital Status

Social Status/Obligations

Travel

Tests/Treatments

Vacation

Violence

Wellness, Change

ILLNESS ORIENTED

GENERAL ILLNESSES

Autoimmune Problems

(*Explanation*: This includes collagen diseases, immunological diseases, blood dyscrasias, and other associated problems.)

Breathing Pattern, Ineffective, **136**
Injury, Potential for, **208**
Self-Care Deficit: Feeding, Bathing/Hygiene, Dressing/Grooming, Toileting, **256**
Skin Integrity, Impairment of: Actual, **279**
Skin Integrity, Impairment of: Potential, **287**
Tissue Perfusion, Alteration in: Cerebral, Cardiopulmonary, Renal, Gastrointestinal, Peripheral, **304**
Urinary Elimination, Alteration in Patterns of, **309**

Cancer

Bowel elimination, Alteration in: Diarrhea, **128**
Coping, Ineffective Individual, **162**
Fear, **176**
Health Maintenance Management, Impaired, **197**
Mobility, Impaired Physical, **221**
Nutrition, Alteration in: Less Than Body Requirements, **227**
Oral Mucous Membrane, Alteration in, **236**
Self-Care Deficit: Feeding, Bathing/Hygiene, Dressing/Grooming, Toileting, **256**
Skin Integrity, Impairment of: Actual, **279**
Skin Integrity, Impairment of: Potential, **287**

Cerebral Vascular Problems

Congenital Abnormalities

Genetic Disorders

Illness, Acute

Illness, Chronic

Illness, Long-Term

Illness, Sudden

Illness, Terminal

ACUTE CARE SETTING

Anesthesia

Chemotherapy

Hospitalization

Tests/Treatments

Tracheostomy

MENTAL HEALTH

Anorexia Nervosa

Bulimia

Catatonia

Delusions

Depression, Severe

Emotional Problems

Violence, Potential for: Self-Directed or Directed at Others, **311**

Hallucinations

Fear, **176**
Health Maintenance, Alteration in, **197**
Self-Care Deficit: Feeding, Bathing/Hygiene, Dressing/ Grooming, Toileting, **256**
Thought Processes, Alteration in, **301**

Mental Illness

Anxiety, **112**
Communication, Impaired Verbal, **148**
Coping, Ineffective Family: Disabling, **158**
Diversional Activity: Deficit, **171**
Grieving, Anticipatory, **189**
Health Maintenance, Alteration in, **197**
Home Maintenance Management, Impaired, **203**
Injury, Potential for, **208**
Mobility, Impaired Physical, **221**
Nutrition, Alteration in: Potential for More Than Body Requirements, **233**
Parenting, Alteration in: Actual or Potential, **242**
Self-Care Deficit: Feeding, Bathing/Hygiene, Dressing/ Grooming, Toileting, **256**
Self-Concept, Disturbance in: Body Image, Self-Esteem, Role Performance, Personal Identity, **263**
Sensory-Perceptual Alteration: Visual, Auditory, Kinesthetic, Gustatory, Tactile, Olfactory, **269**
Sexual Dysfunction, **273**
Skin Integrity, Impairment of: Actual, **279**
Skin Integrity, Impairment of: Potential, **287**
Sleep Pattern Disturbance, **288**
Social Isolation, **292**

Substance Abuse

Social Isolation, **292**
Thought Processes, Alteration in, **301**
Urinary Elimination, Alteration in Patterns, **309**
Violence, Potential for: Self-Directed or Directed at Others, **311**

Suicidal Ideation

Anxiety, **112**
Coping, Ineffective Family: Disabling, **158**
Grieving, Anticipatory, **189**
Grieving, Dysfunctional, **191**
Health Maintenance, Alteration in, **197**
Social Isolation, **292**
Thought Processes, Alteration in, **301**
Violence, Potential for: Self-Directed or Directed at Others, **311**

Withdrawal

Anxiety, **112**
Fear, **176**
Social Isolation, **292**

MOBILITY

Amputation

Anxiety, **112**
Comfort, Alteration in: Pain, **144**
Coping, Ineffective Individual, **162**
Grieving, Anticipatory, **189**
Health Maintenance, Alteration in, **197**
Mobility, Impaired Physical, **221**
Parenting, Alteration in: Actual or Potential, **242**

Self-Care Deficit: Feeding, Bathing/Hygiene, Dressing/
   Grooming, Toileting, **256**
Self-Concept, Disturbance in: Body Image, Self-Esteem,
   Role Performance, Personal Identity, **263**
Sexual Dysfunction, **273**
Social Isolation, **292**

Bedrest

Activity Intolerance, **104**
Activity Intolerance, Potential, **107**
Bowel Elimination, Alteration in: Constipation, **120**
Breathing Pattern, Ineffective, **136**
Coping, Ineffective Individual, **162**
Mobility, Impaired Physical, **221**
Self-Care Deficit: Feeding, Bathing/Hygiene, Dressing/
   Grooming, Toileting, **256**
Sensory-Perceptual Alteration: Visual, Auditory, Kines-
   thetic, Gustatory, Tactile, Olfactory, **269**
Skin Integrity, Impairment of: Actual, **279**
Skin Integrity, Impairment of: Potential, **287**
Spiritual Distress, **298**

Fracture

Comfort, Alteration in: Pain, **144**
Oral Mucous Membrane, Alteration in, **236**
Violence, Potential for: Self-Directed or Directed at Others,
   311

Immobility

Activity Intolerance, **104**
Activity Intolerance, Potential, **107**
Bowel Elimination, Alteration in: Constipation, **120**
Breathing Pattern, Ineffective, **136**

Orthopedic

Paralysis

Comfort, Alteration in: Pain, **144**
Coping, Ineffective Family: Disabling, **158**
Coping, Ineffective Individual, **162**
Grieving, Anticipatory, **189**
Grieving, Dysfunctional, **191**
Health Maintenance, Alteration in, **197**
Home Maintenance Management, Impaired, **203**
Mobility, Impaired Physical, **221**
Noncompliance, **226**
Nutrition, Alteration in: Less Than Body Requirements, **227**
Parenting, Alteration in: Actual or Potential, **242**
Powerlessness, **252**
Self-Care Deficit: Feeding, Bathing/Hygiene, Dressing/ Grooming, Toileting, **256**
Self-Concept, Disturbance in: Body Image, Self-Esteem, Role Performance, Personal Identity, **263**
Sexual Dysfunction, **273**
Skin Integrity, Impairment of: Actual, **279**
Skin Integrity, Impairment of: Potential, **287**
Social Isolation, **292**
Spiritual Distress, **298**
Urinary Elimination, Alteration in Patterns, **309**

Traction

Bowel Elimination, Alteration in: Constipation, **120**
Coping, Ineffective Individual, **162**
Mobility, Impaired Physical, **221**
Sensory-Perceptual Alteration: Visual, Auditory, Kinesthetic, Gustatory, Tactile, Olfactory, **269**

NUTRITION

Fluid and Electrolyte Imbalance

Malnutrition

Nutritional

Total Parenteral Nutrition

PHYSICAL HEALTH

Accidents

Body Defacement

Burns

Confusion

Consciousness, Level of

Cough

Diaphoresis

Mobility, Impaired Physical, **221**
Oral Mucous Membrane, Alteration in, **236**
Skin Integrity, Impairment of: Actual, **279**
Skin Integrity, Impairment of: Potential, **287**
Tissue Perfusion, Alteration in: Cerebral, Cardiopulmonary, Renal, Gastrointestinal, Peripheral, **304**

Diarrhea

Activity Intolerance, **104**
Activity Intolerance, Potential, **107**
Airway Clearance, Ineffective, **108**
Bowel Elimination, Alteration in: Constipation, **120**
Bowel Elimination, Alteration in: Diarrhea, **128**
Breathing Pattern, Ineffective, **136**
Fluid Volume Deficit, Actual (2), **184**
Fluid Volume Deficit, Potential, **185**
Mobility, Impaired Physical, **221**
Nutrition, Alteration in: Less Than Body Requirements, **227**
Oral Mucous Membrane, Alteration in, **236**
Self-Care Deficit: Feeding, Bathing/Hygiene, Dressing/Grooming, Toileting, **256**
Skin Integrity, Impairment of: Actual, **279**
Skin Integrity, Impairment of: Potential, **287**

Fever/Hyperthermia

Activity Intolerance, **104**
Activity Intolerance, Potential, **107**
Breathing Pattern, Ineffective, **136**
Fluid Volume Deficit, Actual (2), **184**
Mobility, Impaired Physical, **221**
Oral Mucous Membrane, Alteration in, **236**
Self-Care Deficit: Feeding, Bathing/Hygiene, Dressing/Grooming, Toileting, **256**

Skin Integrity, Impairment of: Actual, **279**
Skin Integrity, Impairment of: Potential, **287**
Tissue Perfusion, Alteration in: Cerebral, Cardiopulmonary, Renal, Gastrointestinal, Peripheral, **304**

Hemorrhage

Fluid Volume Deficit, Actual (2), **184**
Gas Exchange, Impaired, **186**
Tissue Perfusion, Alteration in: Cerebral, Cardiopulmonary, Renal, Gastrointestinal, Peripheral, **304**

Infection

Airway Clearance, Ineffective, **108**
Bowel Elimination, Alteration in: Diarrhea, **128**
Breathing Pattern, Ineffective, **136**
Gas Exchange, Impaired, **186**
Injury, Potential for, **208**
Nutrition, Alteration in: Less Than Body Requirements, **227**
Oral Mucous Membrane, Alteration in, **236**
Sensory-Perceptual Alteration: Visual, Auditory, Kinesthetic, Gustatory, Tactile, Olfactory, **269**
Skin Integrity, Impairment of: Actual, **279**
Skin Integrity, Impairment of: Potential, **287**
Sleep Pattern Disturbance, **288**
Tissue Perfusion, Alteration in: Cerebral, Cardiopulmonary, Renal, Gastrointestinal, Peripheral, **304**
Urinary Elimination, Alteration in Patterns, **309**

Injury

Bowel Elimination, Alteration in: Constipation, **120**
Breathing Pattern, Ineffective, **136**
Fluid Volume Deficit, Potential, **185**

Self-Care Deficit: Feeding, Bathing/Hygiene, Dressing/
  Grooming, Toileting, **256**
Skin Integrity, Impairment of: Potential, **287**
Violence, Potential for: Self-Directed or Directed at Others,
  311

Pain

Activity Intolerance, **104**
Activity Intolerance, Potential, **107**
Airway Clearance, Ineffective, **108**
Anxiety, **112**
Bowel Elimination, Alteration in: Constipation, **120**
Breathing Pattern, Ineffective, **136**
Coping, Ineffective Family: Compromised, **153**
Coping, Ineffective Individual, **162**
Family Process, Alteration in, **174**
Fear, **176**
Health Maintenance, Alteration in, **197**
Nutrition, Alteration in: Less Than Body Requirements,
  227
Oral Mucous Membrane, Alteration in, **236**
Powerlessness, **252**
Self-Care Deficit: Feeding, Bathing/Hygiene, Dressing/
  Grooming, Toileting, **256**
Spiritual Distress, **298**

Poisoning

Comfort, Alteration in: Pain, **144**
Gas Exchange, Impaired, **186**
Injury, Potential for, **208**
Nutrition, Alteration in: Less Than Body Requirements,
  227
Poisoning: Potential for, **213**

Skin Integrity

Trauma

Vomiting

Cardiopulmonary

Cardiovascular

Ear, Eyes, Nose, Throat

(*Explanation*: This includes all problems associated with the ears, eyes, nose and throat as well as facial structure.)

Endocrine

Gastrointestinal

Genitourinary

Metabolic

ILLNESS/Systems

94

Musculoskeletal

Neurological

Neuromuscular

Peripheral Vascular

(*Explanation*: This includes varicosities, emboli, and other circulatory problems.)

Cardiac Output, Alteration in: Decreased, **142**
Gas Exchange, Impaired, **186**
Sensory-Perceptual Alteration: Visual, Auditory, Kinesthetic, Gustatory, Tactile, Olfactory, **269**
Tissue Perfusion, Alteration in: Cerebral, Cardiopulmonary, Renal, Gastrointestinal, Peripheral, **304**

Renal

Activity Intolerance, **104**
Activity Intolerance, Potential, **107**
Comfort, Alteration in: Pain, **144**
Coping, Ineffective Individual, **162**
Diversional Activity Deficit, **171**
Fluid Volume, Alteration in: Excess, **181**
Fluid Volume Deficit, Actual (1), **183**
Home Maintenance Management, Impaired, **203**
Mobility, Impaired Physical, **221**
Oral Mucous Membrane, Alteration in, **236**
Sexual Dysfunction, **273**
Skin Integrity, Impairment of: Actual, **279**
Skin Integrity, Impairment of: Potential, **287**
Tissue Perfusion, Alteration in: Cerebral, Cardiopulmonary, Renal, Gastrointestinal, Peripheral, **304**
Urinary Elimination, Alteration in Patterns of, **309**

Reproductive

(*Explanation,* : This includes mastectomy, hysterectomy, vasectomy, tubal ligation and other associated problems.)

Anxiety, **112**

Respiratory

(*Explanation*: This includes respiratory diseases, problems, tests, treatments, and procedures.)

SECTION II

NURSING DIAGNOSES

Section II contains the list of approved diagnostic categories according to NANDA. Contents under the categories include definitions, defining characteristics, and nursing diagnoses based on identified etiologies. The accepted etiologies commonly included with each diagnostic category are incorporated in the nursing diagnosis (diagnostic statement). Each nursing diagnosis has a list of related client responses and situations that should be assessed in order to make the identified diagnosis. The client responses and situations are classified according to their association with the state of wellness or illness.

Nursing diagnoses are listed according to each etiology accepted by NANDA. The client responses and situations that are included under the nursing diagnoses are not meant to be all-inclusive or exclusive, but instead are a group of responses and situations that can be used to begin the diagnosing process. The identification of additional data under each nursing diagnosis is expected as the nurse individualizes nursing care in the clinical setting.

Section II can be used separately or in conjunction with Section I, *Index of Nursing Diagnostic Categories*. It may serve as a reference tool for gathering information about nursing diagnoses and related client responses and situations or it may be used to validate assessment data. If it is used for validation, the following process should be utilized:

1. Identify the appropriate diagnostic category by analyzing the definition.
2. Determine whether the collected assessment data correspond with the defining characteristics as listed.
3. Review the nursing diagnoses according to the identified etiologies to locate the desired diagnostic statement.
4. Choose the wellness or illness grouping according to the client data.
5. Examine the client responses and situations in the category to confirm the selection's appropriateness.

II. CONTENTS/Diagnostic Categories

([†]Indicates the author's definition)

([††]Indicates a critical defining characteristic)

DIAGNOSTIC CATEGORY: ACTIVITY INTOLERANCE

Definition: A condition in which the individual is unable to carry out required or desired activities of living.

Defining Characteristics

†† Verbal report of fatigue or weakness
Abnormal heart rate or blood pressure response to activity
Exertional discomfort or dyspnea
Electrocardiographic changes reflecting arrhythmias or ischemia

Nursing Diagnoses Based on Identified Etiologies

Activity Intolerance Related to Bedrest/Immobility
Activity Intolerance Related to Generalized Weakness
Activity Intolerance Related to Sedentary Life Style
Activity Intolerance Related to Imbalance Between Oxygen Supply and Demand

1. ACTIVITY INTOLERANCE RELATED TO BEDREST/ IMMOBILITY

Client Responses and/or Situations Needing Assessment

WELLNESS ORIENTED

Accidents	Fatigue
Casts	Insomnia
Diagnostic Studies	Pregnancy, Late
Dialysis	

ILLNESS ORIENTED

Burns
Cardiopulmonary Disease
Cardiovascular Disease
Hospitalization, Long-Term
Illness, Chronic
Illness, Terminal
Mental Illness, Catatonic
Musculoskeletal Disease

Neurological Disease
Nutritional Deficiencies
Pain
Postoperative Period
Renal Disease
Traction
Trauma

2. ACTIVITY INTOLERANCE RELATED TO GENERALIZED WEAKNESS

Client Responses and/or Situations Needing Assessment

WELLNESS ORIENTED

Agedness
Allergies
Circulation, Decreased

Depression, Moderate
Fatigue
Postpartum Period

ILLNESS ORIENTED

Bedrest, Prolonged
Chemotherapy
Coughing, Severe
Depression, Severe
Diabetes Mellitus
Dialysis
Diaphoresis
Diarrhea
Fever
Fluid and Electrolyte
  Imbalance

Hemorrhage
Hospitalization, Long-Term
Illness, Chronic
Illness, Terminal
Immobility
Metabolic Diseases
Nutritional Deficiencies
Postoperative Period
Radiation Therapy
Respiratory Disease
Vomiting

3. ACTIVITY INTOLERANCE RELATED TO SEDENTARY LIFE STYLE

Client Responses and/or Situations Needing Assessment

WELLNESS ORIENTED

Agedness
Disability
Exercise, Lack of

Malnutrition
Obesity
Retirement

ILLNESS ORIENTED

Depression, Severe
Hospitalization, Long-Term

Illness, Chronic

4. ACTIVITY INTOLERANCE RELATED TO IMBALANCE BETWEEN OXYGEN SUPPLY AND DEMAND

Client Responses and/or Situations Needing Assessment

WELLNESS ORIENTED

Altitude, High
Altitude, Low
Exercise, Overexertion from

ILLNESS ORIENTED

Anxiety, Severe
Bedrest/Immobility, Prolonged

Cardiopulmonary Disease
Cardiovascular Disease
Depression, Severe
Fluid and Electrolyte Imbalance
Nutritional Imbalance
Pain

DIAGNOSTIC CATEGORY:
ACTIVITY INTOLERANCE, POTENTIAL

†*Definition*: (Potential) A condition in which the individual is unable to carry out required or desired activities of living.

Defining Characteristics

History of previous intolerance
Deconditioned status
Presence of circulatory/respiratory problems
Inexperience with the activity

Nursing Diagnoses Based on Identified Etiologies

Potential Activity Intolerance related to (Specify)

1. POTENTIAL ACTIVITY INTOLERANCE RELATED TO (SPECIFY)

††Client Responses and/or Situations Needing Assessment

††See Diagnostic Category: Activity Intolerance

DIAGNOSTIC CATEGORY:
AIRWAY CLEARANCE, INEFFECTIVE

†*Definition:* A condition in which the individual has difficulty in breathing due to partial or complete blockage of the respiratory tract.

Defining Characteristics

Abnormal breath sounds; e.g. rales (crackles), rhonchi (wheezes)

Changes in rate or depth of respiration

Cough, effective/ineffective; with or without sputum

Dyspnea

Tachypnea

Nursing Diagnoses Based on Identified Etiologies

Ineffective Airway Clearance Related to Decreased Energy/Fatigue

Ineffective Airway Clearance Related to Tracheobronchial Infection

Ineffective Airway Clearance Related to Tracheobronchial Obstruction

Ineffective Airway Clearance Related to Tracheobronchial Secretion

Ineffective Airway Clearance Related to Perceptual/Cognitive Impairment

Ineffective Airway Clearance Related to Trauma

1. INEFFECTIVE AIRWAY CLEARANCE RELATED TO DECREASED ENERGY/FATIGUE

Client Responses and/or Situations Needing Assessment

WELLNESS ORIENTED

Altitude, High
Altitude, Low

Depression, Moderate
Exercise, Overexertion from

ILLNESS ORIENTED

Congenital Heart Disease
Congestive Heart Failure
Cough, Chronic
Cystic Fibrosis
Fluid and Electrolyte
   Imbalance
Illness, Prolonged

Level of Consciousness,
   Decreased
Musculoskeletal Disease
Neurological Disease
Pain
Postoperative Period
Respiratory Disease
Vomiting/Diarrhea

2. INEFFECTIVE AIRWAY CLEARANCE RELATED TO TRACHEOBRONCHIAL INFECTION

Client Responses and/or Situations Needing Assessment

ILLNESS ORIENTED

Cough, Chronic
Infection, Ear
Infection, Systemic
Infection, Throat
Laryngitis, Chronic

Pharyngitis, Chronic
Postoperative Period
Post-respirator Period
Respiratory Disease
Trauma

3. INEFFECTIVE AIRWAY CLEARANCE RELATED TO TRACHEOBRONCHIAL OBSTRUCTION

Client Responses and/or Situations Needing Assessment

WELLNESS ORIENTED

Agedness
Aspiration, Food
Aspiration, Foreign Body

Infancy
Newborn

ILLNESS ORIENTED

Congenital Abnormality
Cough, Chronic
Pain, Localized

Trauma
Tumors
Vomiting

4. INEFFECTIVE AIRWAY CLEARANCE RELATED TO TRACHEOBRONCHIAL SECRETION

Client Responses and/or Situations Needing Assessment

WELLNESS ORIENTED

Birth, Breech
Birth, Cesarean

ILLNESS ORIENTED

Anesthesia/Postoperative
Celiac Disease
Congestive Heart Failure

Cough, Inability to
Cough, Ineffective
Cystic Fibrosis

Infant, Isolette
Intermittent Positive Pressure Breathing
Level of Consciousness, Comatose
Level of Consciousness, Decreased
Pneumonia
Postural Drainage
Respiratory Disease
Respiratory Distress Syndrome
Secretions, Pulmonary
Tracheostomy

5. INEFFECTIVE AIRWAY CLEARANCE RELATED TO PERCEPTUAL/COGNITIVE IMPAIRMENT

Client Responses and/or Situations Needing Assessment

WELLNESS ORIENTED

Agedness
Childhood
Infancy

Knowledge Deficit
Mental Retardation

ILLNESS ORIENTED

Level of Consciousness, Comatose
Level of Consciousness, Decreased

6. INEFFECTIVE AIRWAY CLEARANCE RELATED TO TRAUMA

Client Responses and/or Situations Needing Assessment

ILLNESS ORIENTED

Accidents
Cough, Chronic
Coughing (Blood)
Laryngitis
Pain, Localized

Postoperative Period
Post-respirator Period
Voice, Hoarseness
Voice, Raspy

DIAGNOSTIC CATEGORY: ANXIETY

Definition: A vague, uneasy feeling, the source of which is often nonspecific or unknown to the individual.

Defining Characteristics

SUBJECTIVE

Increased tension
Apprehension
Increased helplessness
Uncertainty
Fearful
Scared
Feelings of inadequacy
Shakiness
Fear of unspecific
   consequences
Regretful
Overexcited
Rattled
Distressed
Jittery

OBJECTIVE

††Sympathetic stimulation—
   cardiovascular excitation,
   superficial vasoconstriction,
   pupil dilation
Restlessness
Insomnia
Glancing about
Poor eye contact
Trembling; hand tremors
Extraneous movements—foot
   shuffling; hand, arm
   movements
Expressed concern regarding
   changes in life events
Worried
Anxious
Facial tension
Voice quivering
Focus on self
Increased wariness
Increased perspiration

Nursing Diagnoses Based on Identified Etiologies

Anxiety Related to Unconscious Conflict About Essential Values/Goals of Life

Anxiety Related to Threat to Self-Concept

Anxiety Related to Threat of Death

Anxiety Related to Threat to or Change in Health Status

Anxiety Related to Threat to or Change in Socioeconomic Status

Anxiety Related to Threat to or Change in Role Functioning

Anxiety Related to Threat to or Change in Environment

Anxiety Related to Threat to or Change in Interaction Patterns

Anxiety Related to Situational/Maturational Crises

Anxiety Related to Interpersonal Transmission/Contagion

Anxiety Related to Unmet Needs

1. ANXIETY RELATED TO UNCONSCIOUSNESS CONFLICT ABOUT ESSENTIAL VALUES/ GOALS OF LIFE

Client Responses and/or Situations Needing Assessment

WELLNESS ORIENTED

Abortion

Adolescence

Birth

Culture/Values

Divorce

Education, Change in

Employment, Change in

Employment, Loss of

Habits

Insomnia

Life Style, Change in

Marital Status, Change in

Middle Age

Powerlessness

Pregnancy

Relocation

Retirement
Sleep Pattern, Disturbance in

Spiritual Distress
Young Adulthood

ILLNESS ORIENTED

Alcoholism
Illness, Chronic

Illness, Terminal
Substance Abuse

2. ANXIETY RELATED TO THREAT TO SELF-CONCEPT

See Diagnostic Category: Self-Concept, Disturbance in

Client Responses and/or Situations Needing Assessment

WELLNESS ORIENTED

Abortion
Adolescence
Anorexia/Overeating
Divorce
Economic Status, Change in
Employment, Loss of
Failure, Perceived
Financial Problems
Impotence
Insomnia
Loss, of Loved One
Loss, of Personal Items

Marital Status, Change in
Obesity
Powerlessness
Rape Trauma
Self-Esteem, Lowered
Sexual Dysfunction
Social Isolation
Social Status, Change in
Spiritual Distress
Weight Gain
Weight Loss

ILLNESS ORIENTED

Alcoholism
Amputation
Anorexia Nervosa

Body Defacement
Bulimia
Hysterectomy

Impotence
Mastectomy
Mental Illness, Suicidal
   Ideation
Mental Illness, Withdrawn

Paralysis
Substance Abuse
Tubal Ligation
Vasectomy

3. ANXIETY RELATED TO THREAT OF DEATH

Client Responses and/or Situations Needing Assessment

WELLNESS ORIENTED

Agedness
Diagnostic Studies
Knowledge Deficit
Powerlessness

Self-Esteem, Lowered
Sleep Pattern, Disturbance in
Social Isolation
Spiritual Disturbance

ILLNESS ORIENTED

Cardiovascular Disease,
   Severe
Illness, Terminal
Surgery, Impending

Tests/Treatments, Invasive
Tests/Treatments, Painful
Transplant Surgery,
   Impending

4. ANXIETY RELATED TO THREAT TO OR CHANGE IN HEALTH STATUS

Client Responses and/or Situations Needing Assessment

WELLNESS ORIENTED

Diagnostic Studies
Spiritual Distress
Wellness, Change in Level of

ILLNESS ORIENTED

Diagnosis, New   Illness, Sudden
Illness, Acute   Illness, Terminal
Illness, Chronic

5. ANXIETY RELATED TO THREAT TO OR CHANGE IN SOCIOECONOMIC STATUS

Client Responses and/or Situations Needing Assessment

WELLNESS ORIENTED

Education, Change in   Loss, of Loved One
Education, Graduation   Relocation
Employment, Change in   Retirement

ILLNESS ORIENTED

Hospitalization, Prolonged
Illness, Chronic
Illness, Terminal

6. ANXIETY RELATED TO THREAT TO OR CHANGE IN ROLE FUNCTIONING

Client Responses and/or Situations Needing Assessment

WELLNESS ORIENTED

Depression, Moderate   Family Crisis
Divorce   Family Loss
Employment, Change in   Family Separation
Family Addition   Marital Status, Change in

Powerlessness
Separation
Sexual Dysfunction

Sleep Pattern Disturbance
Social Isolation
Social Obligations

ILLNESS ORIENTED

Hospitalization, Prolonged
Illness, Acute

Illness, Chronic
Illness, Terminal

7. ANXIETY RELATED TO THREAT TO OR CHANGE IN ENVIRONMENT

Client Responses and/or Situations Needing Assessment

WELLNESS ORIENTED

Industry
Pollution, Air
Pollution, Noise

Pollution, Water
Relocation
Weather, Acts of Nature

ILLNESS ORIENTED

Discharge, Early
Hospitalization

Relocation, Intra- or Inter-Agency

8. ANXIETY RELATED TO THREAT TO OR CHANGE IN INTERACTION PATTERNS

Client Responses and/or Situations Needing Assessment

WELLNESS ORIENTED

Adolescence
Agedness

Blindness
Childhood

Consultation, Physician
Deafness
Depression, Moderate
Divorce
Employment, Change in

Infancy
Marital Status, Change in
Separation
Separation, from Loved One
Sexual Dysfunction

ILLNESS ORIENTED

Depression, Severe
Hospitalization
Illness, Acute
Illness, Chronic

Mental Illness
Paralysis
Relocation, Intra- or Inter-Agen

9. ANXIETY RELATED TO SITUATIONAL/MATURATIONAL CRISES

Client Responses and/or Situations Needing Assessment

WELLNESS ORIENTED

Adolescence
Agedness
Childhood
Coping, Ineffective
    (Family)
Coping, Ineffective
    (Individual)
Economic Status,
    Change in
Education, Change in
Employment, Change in
Financial Problems
Infancy

Insomnia
Life Style, Change in
Loss, of Loved One
Loss, of Personal Items
Marital Status, Change in
Middle Age
Powerlessness
Pregnancy
Relocation
Retirement
Sleep Pattern Disturbance
Social Isolation
Social Status, Change in

ILLNESS ORIENTED

Accidents   Illness
Hospitalization   Pain

10. ANXIETY RELATED TO INTERPERSONAL TRANSMISSION/CONTAGION

Client Responses and/or Situations Needing Assessment

WELLNESS ORIENTED

Anxiety, Transmitted   Crisis, of Individual
Crisis, of Community   Crisis, of Loved One
Crisis, of Family

11. ANXIETY RELATED TO UNMET NEEDS

Client Responses and/or Situations Needing Assessment

See Diagnostic Category: Ineffective Individual Coping

WELLNESS ORIENTED

Adolescence   Employment, Change in
Agedness   Financial Problems
Childhood   Incarceration
Death   Infancy
Divorce   Insomnia
Economic Status, Change in   Loss, of Loved One
Education, Change in   Loss, of Personal Items

Marital Status, Change in
Middle Age
Powerlessness
Pregnancy
Relocation
Retirement
Sleep Pattern Disturbance
Social Isolation
Social Obligations
Social Status, Change in
Young Adulthood

ILLNESS ORIENTED

Accidents
Hospitalization
Illness
Illness, Chronic
Illness, Terminal
Pain

DIAGNOSTIC CATEGORY: BOWEL ELIMINATION, ALTERATION IN: CONSTIPATION

†*Definition*: A nonpathological condition in which the individual exhibits infrequent bowel movements or the absence of stool.

Defining Characteristics

Frequency less than usual pattern
Hard-formed stool
Palpable mass
Reported feeling of rectal fullness
Straining at stool
Decreased bowel sounds
Reported feeling of abdominal or rectal fullness or pressure
Less than usual amount of stool
Nausea

Nursing Diagnoses Based on Identified Etiologies

Alteration in Bowel Elimination: Constipation Related to Less Than Adequate Intake

Alteration in Bowel Elimination: Constipation Related to Less Than Adequate Dietary Intake and Bulk

Alteration in Bowel Elimination: Constipation Related to Less Than Adequate Physical Activity or Immobility

Alteration in Bowel Elimination: Constipation Related to Personal Habits

Alteration in Bowel Elimination: Constipation Related to Medications

Alteration in Bowel Elimination: Constipation Related to Chronic Use of Medication and Enemas

Alteration in Bowel Elimination: Constipation Related to Gastrointestinal Obstruction Lesions

Alteration in Bowel Elimination: Constipation Related to Neuromuscular Impairment

Alteration in Bowel Elimination: Constipation Related to Musculoskeletal Impairment

Alteration in Bowel Elimination: Constipation Related to Pain on Defecation

Alteration in Bowel Elimination: Constipation Related to Diagnostic Procedures

Alteration in Bowel Elimination: Constipation Related to Lack of Privacy

Alteration in Bowel Elimination: Constipation Related to Weak Abdominal Muscles

Alteration in Bowel Elimination: Constipation Related to Pregnancy

Alteration in Bowel Elimination: Constipation Related to Emotional Status

1. ALTERATION IN BOWEL ELIMINATION: CONSTIPATION RELATED TO LESS THAN ADEQUATE INTAKE

Client Responses and/or Situations Needing Assessment

WELLNESS ORIENTED

Adolescence
Agedness
Individual, Living Alone
Infant, Breastfeeding

Knowledge Deficit
Life Style, Change
Nutrition, Inadequate

ILLNESS ORIENTED

Alcoholism
Anorexia Nervosa
Bulimia

Malnutrition
Nutrition, T.P.N.
Substance Abuse

2. ALTERATION IN BOWEL ELIMINATION: CONSTIPATION RELATED TO LESS THAN ADEQUATE DIETARY INTAKE AND BULK

Client Responses and/or Situations Needing Assessment

WELLNESS ORIENTED

Childhood
Dental Problems
Dentures, Ill-Fitting
Financial Problems
Infancy
Knowledge Deficit

Nutrition, Carbohydrate
  low
Nutrition, Fiber low
Nutrition, Fluids low
Pregnancy

ILLNESS ORIENTED

Gastroenteritis	Malnutrition
Gastrointestinal Disease	Oral Disease

3. ALTERATION IN BOWEL ELIMINATION: CONSTIPATION RELATED TO LESS THAN ADEQUATE PHYSICAL ACTIVITY OR TO IMMOBILITY

Client Responses and/or Situations Needing Assessment

WELLNESS ORIENTED

Agedness	Life Style, Sedentary
Exercise, Lack of	Middle Age
Fatigue	Obesity
Infancy	

ILLNESS ORIENTED

Bedrest, Prolonged	Neurological Disease
Burns	Paralysis
Cardiopulmonary Disease	Postoperative Period
Cardiovascular Disease	Spinal Cord Injury
Congenital Abnormalities	Spinal Cord Tumors
Depression, Severe	Surgery, Vertebral
Mental Illness, Catatonia	Traction
Musculoskeletal Disease	

4. ALTERATION IN BOWEL ELIMINATION: CONSTIPATION RELATED TO PERSONAL HABITS

Client Responses and/or Situations Needing Assessment

WELLNESS ORIENTED

Child, Holding in by
Elimination, Break in
Routine of

Elimination, Postponing
Laxatives, Excessive Use of

5. ALTERATION IN BOWEL ELIMINATION: CONSTIPATION RELATED TO MEDICATIONS

Client Responses and/or Situations Needing Assessment

WELLNESS ORIENTED

Agedness
Diagnostic Studies
Drugs, Over-the-Counter;
e.g. Iron, Calcium

Drugs, Prescribed
Knowledge Deficit

ILLNESS ORIENTED

Anesthesia
Drug, Barium

Drugs, Prescribed

6. ALTERATION IN BOWEL ELIMINATION: CONSTIPATION RELATED TO CHRONIC USE OF MEDICATION AND ENEMAS

Client Responses and/or Situations Needing Assessment

WELLNESS ORIENTED

Agedness

Knowledge Deficit

ILLNESS ORIENTED

Gastrointestinal Disease

Illness, Chronic

7. ALTERATION IN BOWEL ELIMINATION: CONSTIPATION RELATED TO GASTROINTESTINAL OBSTRUCTIVE LESIONS

Client Responses and/or Situations Needing Assessment

ILLNESS ORIENTED

Diarrhea   Gastrointestinal Disease

8. ALTERATION IN BOWEL ELIMINATION: CONSTIPATION RELATED TO NEUROMUSCULAR IMPAIRMENT

Potential Client Problems and/or Situations Needing Assessment

ILLNESS ORIENTED

Anesthesia   Neurological Disease
Cerebral Palsy   Neuromuscular Disease
Cerebral Vascular Problems   Paralysis
Gastrointestinal Disease   Spinal Cord Injury
Level of Consciousness,   Spinal Cord Lesion
  Comatose
Level of Consciousness,
  Decreased

9. ALTERATION IN BOWEL ELIMINATION: CONSTIPATION RELATED TO MUSCULOSKELETAL IMPAIRMENT

126 **Potential Client Problems and/or Situations Needing Assessment**

ILLNESS ORIENTED

Congenital Abnormalities	Muscular Dystrophy
Megacolon	Musculoskeletal Disease

10. ALTERATION IN BOWEL ELIMINATION: CONSTIPATION RELATED TO PAIN ON DEFECATION

Client Responses and/or Situations Needing Assessment

ILLNESS ORIENTED

Fecal Impaction	Pain, Back
Hemorrhoids	Pilonidal Cyst
Intestinal Fissure	Surgery, Abdominal
Intestinal Obstruction	Surgery, Perineal
Intestinal Tumors	Surgery, Rectal

11. ALTERATION IN BOWEL ELIMINATION: CONSTIPATION RELATED TO DIAGNOSTIC PROCEDURES

Client Responses and/or Situations Needing Assessment

WELLNESS/ILLNESS ORIENTED

Diagnostic Studies, Barium Enema
Diagnostic Studies, Barium Swallow

12. ALTERATION IN BOWEL ELIMINATION: CONSTIPATION RELATED TO LACK OF PRIVACY

Potential Client Problems and/or Situations Needing Assessment

WELLNESS ORIENTED

Employment, Setting of
Family, Crowded Living
School, Setting of

Travel
Vacations

ILLNESS ORIENTED

Hospitalization
Illness, Chronic

Intensive Care Units

13. ALTERATION IN BOWEL ELIMINATION: CONSTIPATION RELATED TO WEAK ABDOMINAL MUSCLES

Potential Client Problems and/or Situations Needing Assessment

ILLNESS ORIENTED

Anorexia Nervosa
Cerebral Vascular Problems
Immobility
Injury, Abdominal
Neurological Disease

Spinal Cord Injury
Spinal Cord Lesions
Spinal Cord Tumors
Surgery, Abdominal

14. ALTERATION IN BOWEL ELIMINATION: CONSTIPATION RELATED TO PREGNANCY

Potential Client Problems and/or Situations Needing Assessment

WELLNESS ORIENTED

Pregnancy

15. ALTERATION IN BOWEL ELIMINATION: CONSTIPATION RELATED TO EMOTIONAL STATUS

Potential Client Problems and/or Situations Needing Assessment

WELLNESS ORIENTED

Child Abuse/Neglect
Crisis, of Family
Crisis, of Individual
Crisis, Maturational

Crisis, Situational
Depression, Moderate
Grieving
Stress/Distress

ILLNESS ORIENTED

Anorexia Nervosa
Bulimia
Depression, Severe

Hospitalization
Medications, Psychotropic

DIAGNOSTIC CATEGORY: BOWEL ELIMINATION, ALTERATION IN: DIARRHEA

†*Definition*: A condition in which the individual has frequent unformed, loose or liquid stools.

Defining Characteristics

Abdominal pain	Increased frequency of
Changes in color	bowel sounds
Cramping	Loose, liquid stools
Increased frequency	Urgency

Nursing Diagnoses Based on Identified Etiologies

Alteration in Bowel Elimination: Diarrhea Related to Stress and Anxiety

Alteration in Bowel Elimination: Diarrhea Related to Dietary Intake

Alteration in Bowel Elimination: Diarrhea Related to Medications

Alteration in Bowel Elimination: Diarrhea Related to Inflammation, Irritation, or Malabsorption

Alteration in Bowel Elimination: Diarrhea Related to Toxins

Alteration in Bowel Elimination: Diarrhea Related to Contaminants

Alteration in Bowel Elimination: Diarrhea Related to Radiation

1. ALTERATION IN BOWEL ELIMINATION: DIARRHEA RELATED TO STRESS AND ANXIETY

Client Responses and/or Situations Needing Assessment

WELLNESS ORIENTED

Adolescence	Child Abuse/Neglect
Agedness	Childhood

Coping, Ineffective Family
Coping, Ineffective Individual
Divorce
Economic Status, Change in
Education, Change in
Employment, Change in
Financial Problems
Insomnia
Loss, of Loved One
Loss, of Personal Items
Marital Status, Change
Relocation
Retirement
Self-Esteem, Lowered
Separation
Social Obligations
Social Status, Change in
Vacation
Wellness, Change in
  Level of

2. ALTERATION IN BOWEL ELIMINATION: DIARRHEA RELATED TO DIETARY INTAKE

Potential Client Problems and/or Situations Needing Assessment

WELLNESS ORIENTED

Allergies, Food
Birth, Premature
Coffee, Increased
  Consumption of
Diet, Starvation
Infancy
Infant, Breastfeeding
Newborn
Diet, Change in
Travel, Change in Food
Travel, Change in Water

ILLNESS ORIENTED

Anorexia Nervosa
Bulimia
Malnutrition
Nutritional Deficiencies
Nutritional Disease

3. ALTERATION IN BOWEL ELIMINATION: DIARRHEA RELATED TO MEDICATIONS

Client Responses and/or Situations Needing Assessment

WELLNESS ORIENTED

Agedness
Allergies
Laxatives, Excessive use of
Medications, Side Effects of
Middle Age

ILLNESS ORIENTED

Antibiotics
Chemotherapy
Illness, Acute
Illness, Chronic
Radiation Therapy

4. ALTERATION IN BOWEL ELIMINATION: DIARRHEA RELATED TO INFLAMMATION, IRRITATION, OR MALABSORPTION

Client Responses and/or Situations Needing Assessment

WELLNESS ORIENTED

Allergies, Food
Diagnostic Studies
Nutrition, Change in Food
Nutrition, High Fiber Foods
Poison, Food
Poisons

ILLNESS ORIENTED

Cancer
Celiac Disease
Diarrhea
Endocrine Disease
Fecal Impaction
Infections
Metabolic Disease
Nutritional Deficiencies

Nutritional Disease

Surgery, Intestinal

Radiation Therapy

5. ALTERATION IN BOWEL ELIMINATION: DIARRHEA RELATED TO TOXINS

Potential Client Problems and/or Situations Needing Assessment

WELLNESS ORIENTED

Poison, Food

Travel, in Native Country

Poison, Toxic

Travel, in Other Countries

ILLNESS ORIENTED

Infection, Bacterial

Infection, Viral

Infection, Parasitic

6. ALTERATION IN BOWEL ELIMINATION: DIARRHEA RELATED TO CONTAMINANTS

Potential Client Problems and/or Situations Needing Assessment

WELLNESS ORIENTED

Poison, Food

Pollution, Water

Poison, Toxic

Travel, Change in Food

Poison, Water

Travel, Change in Water

Pollution, Food

7. ALTERATION IN BOWEL ELIMINATION: DIARRHEA RELATED TO RADIATION

Potential Client Problems and/or Situations Needing Assessment

ILLNESS ORIENTED

Cancer

Radiation, Excessive

X-rays, Excessive

DIAGNOSTIC CATEGORY: BOWEL ELIMINATION, ALTERATION IN: INCONTINENCE

†*Definition*: A condition in which the individual is unable to control the passage of stool.

Defining Characteristics

††Involuntary passage of stool

Nursing Diagnoses Based on Identified Etiologies

Alteration in Bowel Elimination: Incontinence Related to Neuromuscular Involvement

Alteration in Bowel Elimination: Incontinence Related to Musculoskeletal Involvement

Alteration in Bowel Elimination: Incontinence Related to Depression

Alteration in Bowel Elimination: Incontinence Related to Perception or Cognitive Impairment

1. ALTERATION IN BOWEL ELIMINATION: INCONTINENCE RELATED TO NEUROMUSCULAR INVOLVEMENT

134

Potential Client Problems and/or Situations Needing Assessment

WELLNESS ORIENTED

Agedness   Labor
Cough   Pregnancy

ILLNESS ORIENTED

Alcoholism   Neurological Disease
Anesthesia   Neuromuscular Disease
Cerebral Vascular Problems Organic Brain Syndrome
Congenital Abnormalities   Paralysis
Gastrointestinal Disease   Spinal Cord Injury
Level of Consciousness,   Spinal Cord Lesion
  Comatose   Substance Abuse
Level of Consciousness,   Surgery, Gastrointestinal
  Lowered

2. ALTERATION IN BOWEL ELIMINATION: INCONTINENCE RELATED TO MUSCULOSKELETAL INVOLVEMENT

Potential Client Problems and/or Situations Needing Assessment

ILLNESS ORIENTED

Congenital Abnormalities   Paralysis
Musculoskeletal Disease

3. ALTERATION IN BOWEL ELIMINATION: INCONTINENCE RELATED TO DEPRESSION

Client Responses and/or Situations Needing Assessment

WELLNESS ORIENTED

Adolescence
Agedness
Anorexia
Childhood
Divorce
Economic Status, Change in
Employment, Change in
Financial Problems

Insomnia
Loss, of Loved One
Loss, of Personal Items
Marital Status, Change in
Relocation
Retirement
Self-Esteem, Lowered
Separation
Social Status, Change in

ILLNESS ORIENTED

Depression, Severe
Substance Abuse

Trauma, Mental

4. ALTERATION IN BOWEL ELIMINATION: INCONTINENCE RELATED TO PERCEPTION OR COGNITIVE IMPAIRMENT

Client Responses and/or Situations Needing Assessment

WELLNESS ORIENTED

Agedness
Infancy
Knowledge Deficit

Mental Retardation
Newborn

ILLNESS ORIENTED

Alcoholism
Anesthesia

Confusion
Emotional Disorders

Level of Consciousness, Comatose
Level of Consciousness, Low
Organic Brain Syndrome
Substance Abuse

DIAGNOSTIC CATEGORY:
BREATHING PATTERN, INEFFECTIVE

†*Definition*: A condition in which the individual cannot provide sufficient ventilation through normal respirations to maintain body (cellular) functioning.

Defining Characteristics

Dyspnea
Shortness of breath
Tachypnea
Fremitus
Abnormal arterial blood gas
Cyanosis
Cough
Nasal flaring
Respiratory depth change
Assumption of three-point change
Pursed-lip breathing/Prolonged expiratory phase
Increased anteroposterior diameter
Use of accessory muscles
Altered chest excursion

Nursing Diagnoses Based on Identified Etiologies

Ineffective Breathing Pattern Related to Neuromuscular Impairment

Ineffective Breathing Pattern Related to Pain
Ineffective Breathing Pattern Related to Musculoskeletal Impairment
Ineffective Breathing Pattern Related to Perception or Cognitive Impairment
Ineffective Breathing Pattern Related to Anxiety
Ineffective Breathing Pattern Related to Decreased Energy/Fatigue
Ineffective Breathing Pattern Related to Inflammatory Process
Ineffective Breathing Pattern Related to Decreased Lung Expansion
Ineffective Breathing Pattern Related to Tracheobronchial Obstruction

1. INEFFECTIVE BREATHING PATTERN RELATED TO NEUROMUSCULAR IMPAIRMENT

Client Responses and/or Situations Needing Assessment

WELLNESS ORIENTED

Agedness
Birth, Breech

Birth, Cesarean
Birth, Premature

ILLNESS ORIENTED

Anesthesia
Cerebral Palsy
Cerebral Vascular Problems
CNS Depression
Congenital Abnormalities
Level of Consciousness, Comatose

Level of Consciousness, Lowered
Neurological Disease
Neuromuscular Disease
Paralysis
Respiratory Diseases

Respiratory Distress
  Syndrome
Spinal Cord Injury
Spinal Cord Lesion

Substance Abuse
Trauma, Head
Tumor, Cerebral

2. INEFFECTIVE BREATHING PATTERN RELATED TO PAIN

Client Responses and/or Situations Needing Assessment

ILLNESS ORIENTED

Cardiopulmonary Disease
Injury, Back
Respiratory Disease

Surgery, Abdominal
Surgery, Chest
Trauma, Chest

3. INEFFECTIVE BREATHING PATTERN RELATED TO MUSCULOSKELETAL IMPAIRMENT

Client Responses and/or Situations Needing Assessment

WELLNESS ORIENTED

Agedness
Birth, Cesarean

Birth, Premature
Smoking

ILLNESS ORIENTED

Bedrest
Cardiopulmonary Disease
Congenital Abnormalities
Cough, Chronic
Immobility

Musculoskeletal Disease
Respiratory Disease
Substance Abuse
Traction

4. INEFFECTIVE BREATHING PATTERN RELATED TO PERCEPTION OR COGNITIVE IMPAIRMENT

Client Responses and/or Situations Needing Assessment

WELLNESS ORIENTED

Agedness
Childhood
Infancy
Knowledge Deficit

Mental Retardation
Motivation
Noncompliance

ILLNESS ORIENTED

Alcoholism
Anesthesia
Confusion
Emotional Disorders
Level of Consciousness,
  Comatose

Level of Consciousness,
  Decreased
Substance Abuse

5. INEFFECTIVE BREATHING PATTERN RELATED TO ANXIETY

Client Responses and/or Situations Needing Assessment

WELLNESS ORIENTED

Agedness
Coping, Ineffective
  Individual
Crisis, of Family
Crisis, of Individual

Pregnancy
Stress/Distress
Wellness, Change in
  Level of

ILLNESS ORIENTED

Asthma
Cardiopulmonary Disease
Cardiovascular Disease
Diagnosis, New
Emotional Disorders

Pain
Postoperative Period
Tests/Treatments, Invasive
Tests/Treatments, Painful
Trauma

6. INEFFECTIVE BREATHING PATTERN RELATED TO DECREASED ENERGY/FATIGUE

Client Responses and/or Situations Needing Assessment

WELLNESS ORIENTED

Altitude, High
Altitude, Low
Birth, Premature
Birth, Postmature

Depression, Moderate
Exercise, Overexertion from
Nutrition, Starvation Diet
Obesity

ILLNESS ORIENTED

Cardiopulmonary Disease
Cardiovascular Disease
Cough, Chronic
Endocrine Disease
Fever
Fluid and Electrolyte
   Imbalance
Illness, Chronic
Illness, Prolonged
Illness, Terminal

Immunological Disease
Metabolic Disease
Musculoskeletal Disease
Neurological Disease
Nutritional Disease
Pain
Respiratory Disease
Vomiting/Diarrhea

7. INEFFECTIVE BREATHING PATTERN RELATED TO INFLAMMATORY PROCESS

Client Responses and/or Situations Needing Assessment

ILLNESS ORIENTED

Fever
Infection, Lung
Infection, Systemic
Infection, Throat

Respiratory Disease
Respiratory Distress
 Syndrome
Trauma

8. INEFFECTIVE BREATHING PATTERN RELATED TO DECREASED LUNG EXPANSION

Client Responses and/or Situations Needing Assessment

WELLNESS ORIENTED

Allergies
Obesity
Positioning

Posture, Poor
Pregnancy
Smoking

ILLNESS ORIENTED

Asthma
Bedrest, Prolonged
Illness, Terminal
Infection, Lung

Pain
Respiratory Disease
Tumor, Lung

9. INEFFECTIVE BREATHING PATTERN RELATED TO TRACHEOBRONCHIAL OBSTRUCTION

Client Responses and/or Situations Needing Assessment

WELLNESS ORIENTED

Agedness	Childhood
Aspiration, Food	Newborn
Aspiration, Foreign Body	

ILLNESS ORIENTED

Congenital Abnormalities	Secretions, Excessive
Cough, Chronic	Trauma
Infection, Lung	Tumor
Respiratory Disease	

DIAGNOSTIC CATEGORY: CARDIAC OUTPUT, ALTERATION IN: DECREASED

†*Definition*: A condition in an individual in which there is a decrease in circulating blood.

Defining Characteristics

Variations in hemodynamic readings	Rales
	Dyspnea
Arrhythmias; ECG changes	Orthopnea
Fatigue	Restlessness
Jugular vein distension	Change in mental status
Cyanosis; pallor of skin and mucous membranes	Shortness of breath
	Syncope
Oliguria	Vertigo
Decreased peripheral pulses	Edema
Cold, clammy skin	Cough

Frothy sputum
Gallop rhythm, abnormal heart sounds
Weakness

Nursing Diagnoses Based on Identified Etiologies

Alteration in Cardiac Output: Decreased Related to Mechanical

Alteration in Cardiac Output: Decreased Related to Electrical

Alteration in Cardiac Output: Decreased Related to Structural

1. ALTERATION IN CARDIAC OUTPUT: DECREASED RELATED TO MECHANICAL

Client Responses and/or Situations Needing Assessment

ILLNESS ORIENTED

Cardiopulmonary Disease
Cardiovascular Disease
Congestive Heart Failure
Peripheral Vascular Disease

2. ALTERATION IN CARDIAC OUTPUT: DECREASED RELATED TO ELECTRICAL

Client Responses and/or Situations Needing Assessment

ILLNESS ORIENTED

Arrhythmias
Conduction Problems
Congenital Abnormalities
Endocrine Disease
Fluid and Electrolyte Imbalance
Metabolic Disease

3. ALTERATION IN CARDIAC OUTPUT: DECREASED RELATED TO STRUCTURAL

Client Responses and/or Situations Needing Assessment

ILLNESS ORIENTED

Congenital Abnormalities	Trauma, Chest
Scoliosis	Trauma, Heart
Trauma, Airway	Trauma, Lung

DIAGNOSTIC CATEGORY: COMFORT, ALTERATION IN: PAIN

†*Definition*: A condition in which an individual indicates severe discomfort.

Defining Characteristics

SUBJECTIVE	OBJECTIVE
Communication (verbal or coded) of pain descriptors	Guarding behavior—protective Self-focusing
	Narrowed focus; i.e. altered time perception, withdrawal from social contact, impaired thought process
	Distraction behavior; e.g., moaning, crying, pacing, seeking out other people and/or activities, restlessness
	Facial mask of pain; i.e., eyes—lackluster, "beaten look," fixed or scattered movement; grimace

SUBJECTIVE	OBJECTIVE
	Alteration in muscle tone; i.e., may span from listless to rigid
	Autonomic responses; e.g., diaphoresis, blood pressure and pulse increases or decreases, pupillary dilation, increased respiratory rate or decreased (these signs are not seen in chronic stable pain)

Nursing Diagnoses Based on Etiologies

Alteration in Comfort: Pain Related to Biologic Injuring Agents

Alteration in Comfort: Pain Related to Chemical Injuring Agents

Alteration in Comfort: Pain Related to Physical Injuring Agents

Alteration in Comfort: Pain Related to Psychologic Injuring Agents

1. ALTERATION IN COMFORT: PAIN RELATED TO BIOLOGIC INJURING AGENTS

Client Responses and/or Situations Needing Assessment

WELLNESS ORIENTED

Digestive Disorders	Pregnancy
Headache	Skin Disorders
Menstrual Disorders	

ILLNESS ORIENTED

Arthritis	Fracture
Burns	Gastrointestinal Disease
Cardiopulmonary Disease	Musculoskeletal Disease
Cardiovascular Disease	Renal Disease
Contractures	Trauma

2. ALTERATION IN COMFORT: PAIN RELATED TO CHEMICAL INJURING AGENTS

Client Responses and/or Situations Needing Assessment

ILLNESS ORIENTED

Allergies	Poisons
Burns, Caustic	Substance Abuse

3. ALTERATION IN COMFORT: PAIN RELATED TO PHYSICAL INJURING AGENTS

Client Responses and/or Situations Needing Assessment

WELLNESS ORIENTED

Diagnostic Studies	Tests/Treatments

ILLNESS ORIENTED

Electrical Shock	Trauma
Surgery	Venipuncture
Tests/Treatments, Invasive	

4. ALTERATION IN COMFORT: PAIN RELATED TO PSYCHOLOGIC INJURING AGENTS

Client Responses and/or Situations Needing Assessment

WELLNESS ORIENTED

Abortion
Anorexia/Overeating
Bulimia
Child Abuse/Neglect
Crisis, of Individual
Crisis, of Family
Divorce
Economic Status, Change in
Employment, Change in
Failure, Perceived
Family Separation
Financial Problems
Impotence
Incarceration
Insomnia
Loss, of Loved One
Loss, of Personal Items
Marital Status, Change in
Relocation
Retirement
Self-Esteem, Lowered
Social Isolation
Social Status, Change in
Spiritual Distress
Weight Gain
Weight Loss

ILLNESS ORIENTED

Alcoholism
Amputation
Anorexia Nervosa
Body Defacement
Bulimia
Diagnosis, New
Diagnostic Studies
Emotional Disorders
Hospitalization
Illness, Acute
Illness, Chronic
Illness, Terminal
Mastectomy
Paralysis
Substance Abuse
Tubal Ligation
Vasectomy

DIAGNOSTIC CATEGORY: COMMUNICATION, IMPAIRED VERBAL

†*Definition*: A condition in which one is unable to express oneself through speech.

Defining Characteristics

††Unable to speak dominant language
††Does not or cannot speak
 Stuttering; slurring
 Impaired articulation
 Dyspnea
 Disorientation
 Inability to modulate speech
 Inability to find words
 Inability to name words
 Inability to identify objects
 Loose association of ideas
 Flight of ideas
 Incessant verbalization
 Difficulty with phonation
 Inability to speak in sentences

Nursing Diagnoses Based on Identified Etiologies

Impaired Verbal Communication Related to Decrease in Circulation to the Brain
Impaired Verbal Communication Related to Physical Barrier
Impaired Verbal Communication Related to Anatomic Defect
Impaired Verbal Communication Related to Psychologic Barriers

Impaired Verbal Communication Related to Cultural Differences

Impaired Verbal Communication Related to Developmental Stage or Age Rotated

1. IMPAIRED VERBAL COMMUNICATION RELATED TO DECREASE IN CIRCULATION TO THE BRAIN

Client Responses and/or Situations Needing Assessment

WELLNESS ORIENTED

Birth	Coughing
Choking	

ILLNESS ORIENTED

Alcoholism	Substance Abuse
Cardiovascular Disease	Trauma, Face
Cerebral Vascular Problems	Trauma, Head
CNS Depression	Trauma, Neck
Congenital Abnormalities	

2. IMPAIRED VERBAL COMMUNICATION RELATED TO PHYSICAL BARRIER

Client Responses and/or Situations Needing Assessment

ILLNESS ORIENTED

Brain Tumor	Neurological Disease
Dental Problems	Surgery, Oral
Embolus	Tracheostomy
Intubation	

3. IMPAIRED VERBAL COMMUNICATION RELATED TO ANATOMIC DEFECT

Client Responses and/or Situations Needing Assessment

WELLNESS ORIENTED

Ankyloglossia

Blindness

Hearing Loss

Speech Impediment

ILLNESS ORIENTED

Congenital Abnormalities

Disease, Oral

Trauma, Oral

4. IMPAIRED VERBAL COMMUNICATION RELATED TO PSYCHOLOGIC BARRIERS

Client Responses and/or Situations Needing Assessment

See Diagnostic Category: Anxiety

WELLNESS ORIENTED

Anxiety

Fear

Perception, Inaccuracy of

Skin Changes

Stimuli, Lack of

ILLNESS ORIENTED

Mental Illness

Mental Illness, Psychosis

5. IMPAIRED VERBAL COMMUNICATION RELATED TO CULTURAL DIFFERENCES

Client Responses and/or Situations Needing Assessment

WELLNESS ORIENTED

Knowledge Deficit
Language, Barriers to
Language, Foreign
Language, Nonverbal

6. IMPAIRED VERBAL COMMUNICATION RELATED TO DEVELOPMENTAL STAGE OR AGE RELATED

Client Responses and/or Situations Needing Assessment

WELLNESS ORIENTED

Crisis, Agedness-related
Crisis, Adolescence
Crisis, Childhood
Crisis, Infancy
Crisis, Middle Age
Crisis, Young Adulthood
Mental Retardation

DIAGNOSTIC CATEGORY: COPING, FAMILY: POTENTIAL FOR GROWTH

Definition: The family member has effectively managed adaptive tasks involved with the client's health challenge and is exhibiting desire and readiness for enhanced health and growth in regard to self and in relation to the client.

Defining Characteristics

Family members attempt to describe growth impact of crisis on their own values, priorities, goals, or relationships.

Family member is moving in direction of health-promoting and enriching life style which supports and monitors maturational processes, audits and negotiates treatment programs, and generally chooses experiences which optimize wellness.

Individual expresses interest in making contact on a one-to-one basis or on a mutual-aid group basis with another person who has experienced a similar situation.

Degree of independent nursing therapy: High

Nursing Diagnoses Based on Identified Etiologies

(*Explanation*: The person's basic needs are sufficiently gratified and adaptive tasks effectively addressed to enable goals of self-actualization to surface.)

Family Coping Related to Potential for Growth

1. FAMILY COPING RELATED TO POTENTIAL FOR GROWTH

Client Responses and/or Situations Needing Assessment

WELLNESS/ILLNESS ORIENTED

Education
Exercise
Family
Financial Resources

Illness
Individuals Expressed Needed
Support Systems

DIAGNOSTIC CATEGORY:
COPING, INEFFECTIVE FAMILY:
DISABLING

Definition: A usually supportive primary person (family member or close friend) is providing insufficient, ineffective, or compromised support, comfort, assistance, or encouragement which may be needed by the client to manage or master adaptive tasks related to his or her health challenge.

Defining Characteristics

SUBJECTIVE

Client expresses or confirms a concern or complaint about significant other's response to client's health problem

Significant person describes preoccupation with personal reactions, e.g., fear, anticipatory grief, guilt, anxiety, to client's illness, disability, or to other situational or developmental crises

Significant person describes or confirms an inadequate understanding or knowledge base that interferes with effective assistive or supporting behaviors

OBJECTIVE

Significant person attempts assistive or supportive behaviors with less than satisfactory results

Significant person withdraws or enters into limited or temporary personal communication with the client at time of need

Significant person displays protective behavior disproportionate (too little or too much) to the client's abilities or need for autonomy

Degree of independent nursing therapy: High

Comments: Differential diagnosing: The coping strategies of family members addressed in this diagnosis are basically constructive in nature. The constructive but compromised response and intent fall short of their realistic potential for effective situational or crisis management. Changed and refined from previous nursing diagnosis *Coping patterns, ineffective family*.

Nursing Diagnoses Based on Identified Etiologies

Ineffective Family Coping: Compromised Related to Inadequate or Incorrect Information or Understanding by a Primary Person

Ineffective Family Coping: Compromised Related to Temporary Preoccupation by a Significant Person

Ineffective Family Coping: Compromised Related to Temporary Family Disorganization and Role Change

Ineffective Family Coping: Compromised Related to Other Situational or Developmental Crises or Situations the Significant Person May Be Facing

Ineffective Family Coping: Compromised Related to Client Providing Little Support in Turn for the Primary Person

Ineffective Family Coping: Compromised Related to Prolonged Disease or Disability Progression That Exhausts the Supported Capacity of Significant People

1. INEFFECTIVE FAMILY COPING: COMPROMISED RELATED TO INADEQUATE OR INCORRECT INFORMATION OR UNDERSTANDING BY A PRIMARY PERSON

Client Responses and/or Situations Needing Assessment

WELLNESS ORIENTED

Knowledge Deficit

2. INEFFECTIVE FAMILY COPING: COMPROMISED RELATED TO TEMPORARY PREOCCUPATION BY A SIGNIFICANT PERSON

(*Comment*: This person is trying to manage emotional conflicts and personal suffering and is unable to perceive or act effectively in regard to client's needs.)

Client Responses and/or Situations Needing Assessment

WELLNESS ORIENTED

Anxiety, About Change in Interaction Patterns
Anxiety, About Death
Anxiety, About Health Status
Anxiety, About Role Functioning
Anxiety, About Self-Concept
Anxiety, About Socioeconomic Status
Crisis, of Individual
Stress/Distress

3. INEFFECTIVE FAMILY COPING: COMPROMISED RELATED TO TEMPORARY FAMILY DISORGANIZATION AND ROLE CHANGE

Client Responses and/or Situations Needing Assessment

WELLNESS ORIENTED

Crisis, of Family
Crisis, of Individual

Divorce
Education, Change in

Education, Graduation
Employment, Change in
Family, Addition to
Family, Separation in
Loss, of Loved One
Loss, of Personal Items
Marital Status, Change in

Pregnancy
Promotion
Relocation, of Family
Retirement
Separation
Spiritual Distress

4. INEFFECTIVE FAMILY COPING: COMPROMISED RELATED TO OTHER SITUATIONAL OR DEVELOPMENTAL CRISES OR SITUATIONS THE SIGNIFICANT PERSON MAY BE FACING

Client Responses and/or Situations Needing Assessment

WELLNESS ORIENTED

Adolescence
Agedness
Childhood
Divorce
Economic Status, Change
Education, New
Employment, Change in
Family Violence
Financial Problems
Incarceration
Infancy
Loss, of Loved One

Loss, of Personal Items
Marital Status, Change in
Parenting (Childrearing)
Powerlessness
Pregnancy
Relocation
Retirement
Separation
Skin Changes
Social Status, Change in
Spiritual Distress

ILLNESS ORIENTED

Accidents
Hospitalization

Illness
Pain

5. INEFFECTIVE FAMILY COPING: COMPROMISED RELATED TO CLIENT PROVIDING LITTLE SUPPORT IN TURN FOR THE PRIMARY PERSON

Client Responses and/or Situations Needing Assessment

See Diagnostic Category: Coping, Ineffective Individual

WELLNESS ORIENTED

Failure, Perceived	Loss, Personal Items
Loss, Loved One	Self-Esteem, Lowered

ILLNESS ORIENTED

Accidents	Illness
Hospitalization	Pain

6. INEFFECTIVE FAMILY COPING: COMPROMISED RELATED TO PROLONGED DISEASE OR DISABILITY PROGRESSION THAT EXHAUSTS THE SUPPORTED CAPACITY OF SIGNIFICANT PEOPLE

Client Responses and/or Situations Needing Assessment

ILLNESS ORIENTED

Accident	Illness, Chronic
Hospitalization, Long-Term	Illness, Terminal

DIAGNOSTIC CATEGORY: COPING, INEFFECTIVE FAMILY: DISABLING

Definition: The behavior of a significant person (family member or other primary person) disables his or her own capacities and the client's capacities to effectively address tasks essential to either person's adaptation to the health challenge.

Defining Characteristics

Neglectful care of the client in regard to basic human needs and/or illness treatment

Distortion of reality regarding the client's health problem, including extreme denial about its existence or severity

Intolerance

Rejection

Abandonment

Desertion

Carrying on usual routines, disregarding client's needs

Psychosomaticism

Taking on illness signs of client

Decisions and actions by family which are detrimental to economic or social well-being

Agitation, depression, aggression, hostility

Impaired restructuring of a meaningful life for self, impaired individualization, prolonged overconcern for client

Neglectful relationships with other family members

Client's development of helpless, inactive dependence

Degree of independent nursing therapy: Moderate to high

Comments: Regarding the family member's disabling coping response to the client's health challenge, one can describe a family member's response as disabling if it involves short-term coping behaviors which are highly detrimental to the welfare of the client or the significant person. In addition, chronically disabling patterns by a primary person are described as continued use of selected coping skills which have interrupted the person's longer-term capacity to receive, store, or organize information or to react in regard to it. This diagnosis is changed and refined from previous nursing diagnosis *Coping, ineffective family*.

Nursing Diagnoses Based on Identified Etiologies

Ineffective Family Coping: Disabling Related to Significant Person with Chronically Unexpected Feelings of Guilt, Hostility, Despair

Ineffective Family Coping: Disabling Related to Dissonant Discrepancy of Coping Styles

Ineffective Family Coping: Disabling Related to Highly Ambivalent Family Relationships

Ineffective Family Coping: Disabling Related to Arbitrary Handling of a Family's Resistance to Treatment

1. INEFFECTIVE FAMILY COPING: DISABLING RELATED TO SIGNIFICANT PERSON WITH CHRONICALLY UNEXPECTED FEELINGS OF GUILT, HOSTILITY, DESPAIR

Client Responses and/or Situations Needing Assessment

WELLNESS ORIENTED

Abortion	Crisis, of Individual
Anxiety	Despair

160

Divorce
Economic Status, Change in
Employment, Change in
Failure, Perceived
Family Separation
Fear
Financial Problems
Guilt
Hostility
Impotence

Loss, of Loved One
Loss, of Personal Items
Marital Status, Change in
Rape Trauma
Relocation, of Family
Self-Esteem, Lowered
Separation
Sexual Dysfunction
Social Status, Change in
Stress/Distress

ILLNESS ORIENTED

Alcoholism
Body Defacement
Depression, Severe
Hospitalization
Illness, Chronic
Illness, Terminal

Mastectomy
Mental Illness, Paranoia
Mental Illness, Suicidal
   Ideation
Paralysis
Substance Abuse

2. INEFFECTIVE FAMILY COPING: DISABLING RELATED TO DISSONANT DISCREPANCY OF COPING STYLES

Comment: This is a discrepancy in coping styles being used to deal with adaptive tasks by the significant person and client or among significant people.

Client Responses and/or Situations Needing Assessment

WELLNESS ORIENTED

Crisis, of Family
Crisis, of Individual

Employment, Change in
Family Separation

Financial Problems
Impotence
Infertility
Knowledge Deficit
Loss, of Loved One

Marital Status, Change in
Sexual Dysfunction
Social Status, Change in
Stress/Distress

ILLNESS ORIENTED

Diagnosis, New
Emotional Disorders
Hospitalization, Long-Term
Illness, Acute

Illness, Chronic
Illness, Sudden
Illness, Terminal

3. INEFFECTIVE FAMILY COPING: DISABLING RELATED TO HIGHLY AMBIVALENT FAMILY RELATIONSHIPS

Client Responses and/or Situations Needing Assessment

WELLNESS ORIENTED

Abortion
Crisis, of Family
Crisis, of Individual
Divorce
Economic Status, Change in
Employment, Change in
Family Separation

Financial Problems
Loss, of Loved One
Marital Status, Change in
Middle Age
Separation
Social Status, Change in

ILLNESS ORIENTED

Diagnosis, New
Hospitalization, Long-Term
Illness, Acute
Illness, Chronic

Illness, Sudden
Illness, Terminal
Mental Illness

4. INEFFECTIVE FAMILY COPING: DISABLING RELATED TO ARBITRARY HANDLING OF A FAMILY'S RESISTANCE TO TREATMENT

(*Explanation*: This tends to solidify defensiveness as it fails to deal adequately with underlying anxiety.)

Client Responses and/or Situations Needing Assessment

WELLNESS ORIENTED

Anxiety   Stress/Distress
Noncompliance, with Treatment

DIAGNOSTIC CATEGORY: COPING, INEFFECTIVE INDIVIDUAL

† *Definition*: Ineffective coping is the impairment of adaptive behaviors and problem-solving abilities.

Defining Characteristics

†† Verbalization of inability to cope or inability to ask for help
Inability to meet role expectations
Inability to meet basic needs
†† Inability to problem-solve
Destructive behavior toward self or others
Inappropriate use of defense mechanisms

Change in usual communication patterns
Verbal manipulation
High illness rate
High rate of accidents
Overeating
Lack of appetite
Excessive smoking
Excessive drinking
Overuse of prescribed tranquilizers
Alcohol proneness
High blood pressure
Chronic fatigue
Insomnia
Muscular tension
Ulcers
Frequent headaches
Frequent neckaches
Irritable bowel
Chronic worry
General irritability
Poor self-esteem
Chronic anxiety
Emotional tension
Chronic depression

Nursing Diagnoses Based on Identified Etiologies

Ineffective Individual Coping Related to Situational Crises

Ineffective Individual Coping Related to Maturational Crises

Ineffective Individual Coping Related to Personal Vulnerability

Ineffective Individual Coping Related to Multiple Life Changes

Ineffective Individual Coping Related to No Vacations

Ineffective Individual Coping Related to Inadequate Relaxation

Ineffective Individual Coping Related to Inadequate Support Systems

Ineffective Individual Coping Related to Little or No Exercise

Ineffective Individual Coping Related to Poor Nutrition

Ineffective Individual Coping Related to Unmet Expectations

Ineffective Individual Coping Related to Work Overload

Ineffective Individual Coping Related to Too Many Deadlines

Ineffective Individual Coping Related to Unrealistic Perceptions

Ineffective Individual Coping Related to Inadequate Coping Method

1. INEFFECTIVE INDIVIDUAL COPING RELATED TO SITUATIONAL CRISES

Client Responses and/or Situations Needing Assessment

WELLNESS ORIENTED

Accidents
Anorexia/Overeating
Child Abuse/Neglect
Divorce
Economic Status, Change in
Education, Change in
Employment, Change in
Financial Problems
Incarceration
Loss, of Loved One
Loss, of Personal Items
Powerlessness
Rape Trauma
Self-Concept, Disturbance of
Separation
Sleep Pattern Disturbance
Social Isolation
Social Obligations
Social Status, Change in
Spiritual Distress

ILLNESS ORIENTED

Accidents
Hospitalization
Illness
Pain

2. INEFFECTIVE INDIVIDUAL COPING RELATED TO MATURATIONAL CRISES

Client Responses and/or Situations Needing Assessment

WELLNESS ORIENTED

Adolescence
Agedness
Childhood
Crisis, Empty Nest
Crisis, Midlife
Divorce
Education

Infancy
Marriage, New
Parenting (Childrearing)
Pregnancy
Retirement
Separation

3. INEFFECTIVE INDIVIDUAL COPING RELATED TO PERSONAL VULNERABILITY

Client Responses and/or Situations Needing Assessment

WELLNESS ORIENTED

Anorexia/Overeating
Child Abuse/Neglect
Divorce
Economic Status, Change in
Employment, Change in
Failure, Perceived
Financial Loss
Financial Problems
Impotence
Insomnia
Loss, of Loved One

Loss, of Personal Items
Marital Status, Change in
Powerlessness
Rape Trauma
Relocation
Self-Esteem, Lowered
Separation
Sleep Pattern Disturbance
Social Status, Change in
Weight Gain
Weight Loss

ILLNESS ORIENTED

Alcoholism
Amputation

Body Defacement
Emotional Disorders

Hysterectomy	Substance Abuse
Immobility	Tubal Ligation
Mastectomy	Vasectomy
Paralysis	

4. INEFFECTIVE INDIVIDUAL COPING RELATED TO MULTIPLE LIFE CHANGES

Client Responses and/or Situations Needing Assessment

See Diagnostic Category: Anxiety

WELLNESS ORIENTED

Crisis, Community	Marital Status, Change in
Crisis, of Family	Powerlessness
Crisis, of Individual	Pregnancy
Divorce	Relocation
Economic Status, Change in	Retirement
Employment, Change in	Separation
Financial Problems	Sleep Pattern Disturbance
Incarceration	Social Isolation
Loss, of Loved One	Social Status, Change in
Loss, of Personal Items	Spiritual Distress

5. INEFFECTIVE INDIVIDUAL COPING RELATED TO NO VACATIONS

Client Responses and/or Situations Needing Assessment

See Diagnostic Category: Anxiety

WELLNESS ORIENTED

Anxiety	Economic Status, Change in
Crisis, of Family	Emotions, Change in

Employment, Change in
Financial Problems

Insomnia
Stress/Distress

ILLNESS ORIENTED

Cardiopulmonary Disease
Gastrointestinal Disease

Hypertension

6. INEFFECTIVE INDIVIDUAL COPING RELATED TO INADEQUATE RELAXATION

Client Responses and/or Situations Needing Assessment

See Diagnostic Category: Anxiety

WELLNESS ORIENTED

Anxiety
Crisis, of Family
Crisis, of Individual
Economic Status, Change in

Employment, Change in
Financial Problems
Sleep Pattern Disturbance
Stress/Distress

ILLNESS ORIENTED

Cardiopulmonary Disease
Gastrointestinal Disease

Hypertension
Migraine Headache

7. INEFFECTIVE INDIVIDUAL COPING RELATED TO INADEQUATE SUPPORT SYSTEMS

Client Responses and/or Situations Needing Assessment

See Diagnostic Category: Anxiety

WELLNESS ORIENTED

Distant Family   Social Isolation
Loss, of Loved One

ILLNESS ORIENTED

Emotional Disorders   Isolation, Hospital

8. INEFFECTIVE INDIVIDUAL COPING RELATED TO LITTLE OR NO EXERCISE

Client Responses and/or Situations Needing Assessment

See Diagnostic Category: Anxiety

WELLNESS ORIENTED

Agedness   Obesity
Life Style, Sedentary   Retirement

ILLNESS ORIENTED

Bedrest   Illness, Prolonged
Cancer   Immobility
Cardiopulmonary Disease   Musculoskeletal Disease
Cardiovascular Disease   Neurological Disease
Dialysis   Renal Disease
Hospitalization, Long-Term   Traction
Illness, Chronic   Trauma

9. INEFFECTIVE INDIVIDUAL COPING RELATED TO POOR NUTRITION

Client Responses and/or Situations Needing Assessment

See Diagnostic Category: Anxiety

WELLNESS ORIENTED

Abuse
Adolescence
Agedness
Childhood
Dental Problems
Dentures, Ill-Fitting

Financial Problems
Infancy
Knowledge Deficit
Life Style, Change in
Obesity

ILLNESS ORIENTED

Anorexia Nervosa
Bulimia
Fluid and Electrolyte
   Imbalance

Gastroenteritis
Gastrointestinal Disease
Oral Disease
Malnutrition

10. INEFFECTIVE INDIVIDUAL COPING RELATED TO UNMET EXPECTATIONS

Client Responses and/or Situations Needing Assessment

See Diagnostic Category: Anxiety

WELLNESS ORIENTED

Adolescence
Death, Impending
Divorce
Education, Change in
Employment, Change in
Insomnia
Marital Status, Change in
Middle Age
Parenting (Childrearing)
Powerlessness

Pregnancy
Relocation
Retirement
Separation
Sleep Pattern Disturbance
Social Isolation
Social Obligations
Spiritual Distress
Young Adulthood

ILLNESS ORIENTED

Illness, Chronic   Illness, Terminal

11. INEFFECTIVE INDIVIDUAL COPING RELATED TO WORK OVERLOAD

Client Responses and/or Situations Needing Assessment

See Diagnostic Category: Anxiety

WELLNESS ORIENTED

Anxiety   Fatigue
Crisis, of Family   Financial Problems
Crisis, of Individual   Sleep Pattern Disturbance
Economic Status, Change in Social Isolation
Employment, Change in   Stress/Distress

12. INEFFECTIVE INDIVIDUAL COPING RELATED TO TOO MANY DEADLINES

Client Responses and/or Situations Needing Assessment

See Diagnostic Category: Anxiety

WELLNESS ORIENTED

Anxiety   Financial Problems
Crisis, of Family   Stress/Distress
Crisis, of Individual   Stress, Family-Related
Economic Status, Change   Stress, Work-Related
  in
Employment, Change in

13. INEFFECTIVE INDIVIDUAL COPING RELATED TO UNREALISTIC PERCEPTIONS

Client Responses and/or Situations Needing Assessment

See Diagnostic Category: Anxiety

WELLNESS ORIENTED

Knowledge Deficit

14. INEFFECTIVE INDIVIDUAL COPING RELATED TO INADEQUATE COPING METHOD

Client Responses and/or Situations Needing Assessment

See Diagnostic Category: Anxiety

WELLNESS ORIENTED

Childhood
Crisis, of Family
Crisis, of Individual
Emotions

Infancy
Knowledge Deficit
Support Systems, Lack of

DIAGNOSTIC CATEGORY: DIVERSIONAL ACTIVITY DEFICIT

†*Definition*: A condition in which the individual has a decrease in recreational activities and leisure time.

Defining Characteristics

Client's statements regarding the following:
Boredom

Wish there were something to do, to read, etc.
Usual hobbies cannot be undertaken in hospital

Nursing Diagnoses Based on Identified Etiologies

Diversional Activity Deficit Related to Environmental Lack of Diversional Activities

Diversional Activity Deficit Related to Long-Term Hospitalization

Diversional Activity Deficit Related to Frequently Lengthy Treatments

Diversional Activity Deficit Related to Life Changes

1. DIVERSIONAL ACTIVITY DEFICIT RELATED TO ENVIRONMENTAL LACK OF DIVERSIONAL ACTIVITIES

Client Responses and/or Situations Needing Assessment

WELLNESS ORIENTED

Financial Problems
Incarceration

Mental Retardation
Retirement

ILLNESS ORIENTED

Hospitalization, Prolonged

2. DIVERSIONAL ACTIVITY DEFICIT RELATED TO LONG-TERM HOSPITALIZATION

Client Responses and/or Situations Needing Assessment

ILLNESS ORIENTED

Cerebral Vascular Problems
Illness, Chronic
Illness, Terminal

Mental Illness
Trauma, Multiple

3. DIVERSIONAL ACTIVITY DEFICIT RELATED TO FREQUENTLY LENGTHY TREATMENTS

Client Responses and/or Situations Needing Assessment

ILLNESS ORIENTED

Chemotherapy
Dialysis

Hyperalimentation

4. DIVERSIONAL ACTIVITY DEFICIT RELATED TO LIFE CHANGES

Client Responses and/or Situations Needing Assessment

See Diagnostic Category: Anxiety

WELLNESS ORIENTED

Crisis, of Family
Crisis, of Individual
Divorce
Economic Status, Change in
Education
Employment, Change in
Financial Problems
Incarceration
Loss, of Loved One
Loss, of Personal Items

Marital Status, Change in
Marriage, New
Middle Age
Pregnancy
Retirement
Separation
Social Status, Change in
Wellness, Change in
    Level of
Young Adulthood

DIAGNOSTIC CATEGORY: FAMILY PROGRESS, ALTERATION IN

†*Definition:* A condition in which a healthy family is unable to carry out the tasks and functions of the family unit.

Defining Characteristics

Family system unable to meet physical needs for its members

Family system unable to meet emotional needs of its members

Family system unable to meet spiritual needs of its members

Parents do not demonstrate respect for each other's views on childrearing practices

Inability to express or accept wide range of feelings

Inability to express or accept feelings of members

Inability to accept or receive help appropriately

Family unable to meet security needs of its members

Inability of family members to relate to each other for mutual growth and maturation

Family uninvolved in community activities

Rigidity in function and roles

Family does not demonstrate respect for individuality and autonomy of its members

Family inability to adapt to change or to deal with traumatic experience constructively

Family fails to accomplish current or past developmental task

Ineffective family decision-making process

Failure to send and receive clear messages

Inappropriate boundary maintenance

Inappropriate or poorly communicated family rules, rituals, symbols
Unexamined family myths
Inappropriate level and direction of energy

Nursing Diagnoses Based on Identified Etiologies

Alteration in Family Process Related to Situational Transition and/or Crises
Alteration in Family Process Related to Developmental Transition and/or Crises

1. ALTERATION IN FAMILY PROCESS RELATED TO SITUATIONAL TRANSITION AND/OR CRISES

Client Responses and/or Situations Needing Assessment

WELLNESS ORIENTED

Accidents
Adolescence
Divorce
Economic Status, Change in
Education, Change in
Employment, Change in
Employment, Loss of
Family Violence
Financial Problems
Incarceration

Loss, of Loved One
Loss, of Personal Items
Marital Status, Change in
Middle Age
Rape Trauma
Relocation
Separation
Social Status, Change in
Spiritual Distress
Travel

ILLNESS ORIENTED

Accidents
Hospitalization

Illness
Pain

2. ALTERATION IN FAMILY PROCESS RELATED TO DEVELOPMENTAL TRANSITION AND/OR CRISES

Client Responses and/or Situations Needing Assessment

WELLNESS ORIENTED

Adolescence
Agedness
Childhood
Divorce
Education, Change in
Infancy
Marital Status, Change in

Middle Age
Parenting (Childrearing)
Pregnancy
Retirement
Separation
Young Adulthood

DIAGNOSTIC CATEGORY: FEAR

Definition: Fear is a feeling of dread related to an identifiable source which the person validates.

Defining Characteristics

SUBJECTIVE	OBJECTIVE
Increased tension	Increased alertness
Apprehension	Concentration on source
Impulsiveness	Wide-eyed
Decreased self-assurance	Attack behavior
Afraid	Focus on "it, out there"
Scared	Fight behavior—aggressive
Terrified	Flight behavior—withdrawal
Panic	Sympathetic stimulation—
Frightened	cardiovascular excitation,
Jittery	superficial vasoconstriction,
	pupil dilation

Nursing Diagnoses Based on Identified Etiologies

Fear Related to Natural or Innate Origins
Fear Related to Learned Response
Fear Related to Separation from Support System in a Potentially Threatening Situation
Fear Related to Knowledge Deficit or Unfamiliarity
Fear Related to Language Barriers
Fear Related to Sensory Impairment
Fear Related to Phobic Stimulus or Phobia
Fear Related to Environmental Stimuli

1. FEAR RELATED TO NATURAL OR INNATE ORIGINS

Client Responses and/or Situations Needing Assessment

WELLNESS ORIENTED

Anxiety	Pregnancy, Labor
Death	Sudden Noise
Height	Weather, Acts of Nature
Loss, of Physical Support	

ILLNESS ORIENTED

Death, Impending	Illness, Terminal
Illness	Pain

2. FEAR RELATED TO LEARNED RESPONSE

(*Comment*: This diagnosis is the result of conditioning, modeling from, or identification with others.)

Client Responses and/or Situations Needing Assessment

WELLNESS ORIENTED

Adolescence	Middle Age
Agedness	Stress/Distress
Childhood	Young Adulthood

ILLNESS ORIENTED

Anesthesia	Disease
Cancer	Surgery
Death	

3. FEAR RELATED TO SEPARATION FROM SUPPORT SYSTEM IN A POTENTIALLY THREATENING SITUATION

Client Responses and/or Situations Needing Assessment

WELLNESS ORIENTED

Crisis, of Family	Marital Status, Change in
Diagnostic Studies	Relocation
Distant Family	Separation
Divorce	Skin Changes
Family Separation	Spiritual Distress
Incarceration	Tests/Treatments

ILLNESS ORIENTED

Diagnostic Studies	Tests/Treatments, Invasive
Hospitalization	Tests/Treatments, Painful

4. FEAR RELATED TO KNOWLEDGE DEFICIT OR UNFAMILIARITY

Client Responses and/or Situations Needing Assessment

WELLNESS ORIENTED

Anxiety
Childhood, Developmental
  Tasks of

Diagnostic Studies
Parenting (Childrearing)
Stress/Distress

ILLNESS ORIENTED

Diagnosis, New
Diagnostic Studies

Hospitalization

5. FEAR RELATED TO LANGUAGE BARRIERS

Client Responses and/or Situations Needing Assessment

WELLNESS ORIENTED

Blindness
Cultural Barriers
Hearing Loss
Language, Foreign

Language, Nonverbal
Speech Impediment
Terminology, Different

6. FEAR RELATED TO SENSORY IMPAIRMENT

Client Responses and/or Situations Needing Assessment

WELLNESS ORIENTED

Anxiety
Blindness

Hearing Loss
Speech Impediment

ILLNESS ORIENTED

Cerebral Vascular Problems
CNS Depression
Congenital Abnormalities
Hallucinations
Neurological Disease
Spinal Cord Injury

Substance Abuse
Surgery, Ear
Surgery, Eye
Surgery, Oral
Trauma, Face
Trauma, Head

7. FEAR RELATED TO PHOBIC STIMULUS OR PHOBIA

Client Responses and/or Situations Needing Assessment

WELLNESS ORIENTED

Agedness
Childhood
Infancy

Middle Age
Young Adulthood

ILLNESS ORIENTED

Mental Illness, Phobias

Mental Illness, Withdrawal

8. FEAR RELATED TO ENVIRONMENTAL STIMULI

Client Responses and/or Situations Needing Assessment

WELLNESS ORIENTED

Employment, Change in
Incarceration

Relocation
Tests/Treatments

ILLNESS ORIENTED

Anesthesia

Hospitalization

Illness, Sudden   Surgery
Illness, Terminal   Tests/Treatments

DIAGNOSTIC CATEGORY: FLUID VOLUME, ALTERATION IN: EXCESS

†*Definition*: A condition in which the individual has an increase in body fluids.

Defining Characteristics

Edema
Effusion
Anasarca
Weight gain
Shortness of breath, orthopnea
Intake greater than output
Third heart sound
Pulmonary congestion on x-ray film
Abnormal breath sounds: crackles (rales)
Change in respiratory sound
Change in mental status
Decreased hemoglobin, hematocrit
Blood pressure changes
Central venous pressure changes
Pulmonary artery pressure changes
Jugular venous distinction
Positive hepatojugular reflex
Oliguria
Specific gravity changes
Azoturia
Altered electrolytes
Restlessness and anxiety

182 ## Nursing Diagnoses Based on Identified Etiologies

Alteration in Fluid Volume: Excess Related to Compromised Regulatory Mechanism

Alteration in Fluid Volume: Excess Related to Excess Fluid Intake

Alteration in Fluid Volume: Excess Related to Excess Sodium Intake

1. ALTERATION IN FLUID VOLUME: EXCESS RELATED TO COMPROMISED REGULATORY MECHANISM

Client Responses and/or Situations Needing Assessment

ILLNESS ORIENTED

Cardiopulmonary Disease
Cardiovascular Disease
Endocrine Disease

Metabolic Disease
Renal Disease

2. ALTERATION IN FLUID VOLUME: EXCESS RELATED TO EXCESS FLUID INTAKE

Client Responses and/or Situations Needing Assessment

ILLNESS ORIENTED

Alcoholism
Malnutrition
Nutrition, TPN

Parenteral Therapy
Water Intoxication

3. ALTERATION IN FLUID VOLUME: EXCESS RELATED TO EXCESS SODIUM INTAKE

Client Responses and/or Situations Needing Assessment

WELLNESS ORIENTED

Nutrition, Increased Sodium Intake

ILLNESS ORIENTED

Cardiovascular Disease   Metabolic Disease
Endocrine Disease   Renal Disease

DIAGNOSTIC CATEGORY: FLUID VOLUME DEFICIT, ACTUAL (1)

†*Definition*: A condition in which the individual has a decrease in body fluids.

Defining Characteristics

Dilute urine   Increased body temperature
Increased urine output   Dry skin
Sudden weight loss   Dry mucous membranes
Possible weight gain   Hemoconcentration
Hypotension   Weakness
Decreased venous filling   Edema
Increased pulse rate   Thirst
Decreased skin turgor
Decreased pulse volume
    and pressure

Nursing Diagnoses Based on Identified Etiologies

Actual Fluid Volume Deficit Related to Failure of Regulatory Mechanisms

1. ACTUAL FLUID VOLUME DEFICIT RELATED TO FAILURE OF REGULATORY MECHANISMS

Potential Client Problems and/or Situations Needing Assessment

ILLNESS ORIENTED

Cardiopulmonary Disease   Metabolic Disease
Cardiovascular Disease   Renal Disease
Endocrine Disease

DIAGNOSTIC CATEGORY: FLUID VOLUME DEFICIT, ACTUAL (2)

†*Definition:* A condition in which the individual has a decrease in body fluids.

Defining Characteristics

Decreased urine output   Decreased skin turgor
Concentrated urine   Decreased pulse volume and
Output greater than intake   pressure
Sudden weight loss   Change in mental state
Decreased venous filling   Increased body tempeature
Hemoconcentration   Dry Skin
Increased serum sodium   Dry mucous membranes
Hypotension   Weakness
Thirst

Nursing Diagnoses Based on Identified Etiologies

Actual Fluid Volume Deficit Related to Active Loss

1. ACTUAL FLUID VOLUME DEFICIT RELATED TO ACTIVE LOSS

Client Responses and/or Situations Needing Assessment

ILLNESS ORIENTED

Burns
Dehydration
Dialysis
Diaphoresis
Diarrhea
Endocrine Disease

Hemorrhage
Hyperthermia
Metabolic Disease
Respiratory, Hyperpnea
Respiratory, Hyperventilation
Vomiting

DIAGNOSTIC CATEGORY: FLUID VOLUME DEFICIT, POTENTIAL

†*Definition*: (Potential) A condition in which the individual has a decrease in body fluids.

Defining Characteristics

Increased fluid output
Urinary frequency

Thirst
Altered Intake

Nursing Diagnoses Based on Identified Etiologies

Potential Fluid Volume Deficit Related to Extremes of Age

1. POTENTIAL FLUID VOLUME DEFICIT RELATED TO EXTREMES OF AGE

Client Responses and/or Situations Needing Assessment

WELLNESS ORIENTED

Age, Extremes of
Knowledge Deficit, Related to Fluid Volume
Medications (diuretics)
Weight, Extremes of

ILLNESS ORIENTED

Deviations affecting access to, intake of, or absorption of
    fluids, e.g., physical activity
Excessive losses through normal routes, e.g., diarrhea
Factors influencing fluid needs, e.g., hypermetabolic states
Loss of fluid through abnormal routes, e.g., indwelling
    tubes

DIAGNOSTIC CATEGORY: GAS EXCHANGE, IMPAIRED

†*Definition:* A condition in which the individual has impaired respiratory function.

Defining Characteristics

Confusion
Somnolence
Restlessness
Irritability

Inability to move secretions
Hypercapnea
Hypoxia

Nursing Diagnoses Based on Identified Etiologies

Impaired Gas Exchange Related to Altered Oxygen Supply
Impaired Gas Exchange Related to Alveolar-Capillary Membrane Changes
Impaired Gas Exchange Related to Altered Blood Flow
Impaired Gas Exchange Related to Altered Oxygen-Carrying Capacity of Blood

1. IMPAIRED GAS EXCHANGE RELATED TO ALTERED OXYGEN SUPPLY

Client Responses and/or Situations Needing Assessment

WELLNESS ORIENTED

Agedness	Cough, Chronic
Altitude, High	Exercise, Overexertion from
Altitude, Low	Hyperventilation
Birth, Premature	Newborn
Choking	

ILLNESS ORIENTED

Cardiopulmonary Disease	Congenital Abnormalities
Cardiovascular Disease	Peripheral Vascular Disease

2. IMPAIRED GAS EXCHANGE RELATED TO ALVEOLAR-CAPILLARY MEMBRANE CHANGES

Client Responses and/or Situations Needing Assessment

WELLNESS ORIENTED

Agedness	Allergies

Birth, Premature   Poison

ILLNESS ORIENTED

Allergies   Respiratory Disease
Congenital Abnormalities   Respiratory Distress
Infection, Lung   Syndrome
Poison   Surgery

3. IMPAIRED GAS EXCHANGE RELATED TO ALTERED BLOOD FLOW

Client Responses and/or Situations Needing Assessment

ILLNESS ORIENTED

Arrhythmias   Congenital Abnormalities
Cardiopulmonary Disease   Congestive Heart Failure
Cardiovascular Disease

4. IMPAIRED GAS EXCHANGE RELATED TO ALTERED OXYGEN-CARRYING CAPACITY OF BLOOD

Client Responses and/or Situations Needing Assessment

ILLNESS ORIENTED

Anemia   Respiratory Disease
Burns   Respiratory Distress
Dehydration   Syndrome
Hemorrhage
Poisoning, Carbon
   Monoxide

DIAGNOSTIC CATEGORY: GRIEVING, ANTICIPATORY

Definition: A condition in which the individual grieves before an actual loss.

Defining Characteristics

Potential loss of significant object
Expression of distress at potential loss
Denial of potential loss
Guilt
Anger
Sorrow
Choked feelings
Changes in eating habits
Alterations in sleep patterns
Alterations in activity level
Altered libido
Altered communication patterns

Nursing Diagnoses Based on Identified Etiologies

Anticipatory Grieving Related to Perceived Potential Loss of Significant Other
Anticipatory Grieving Related to Perceived Potential Loss of Physiopsychosocial Well-Being
Anticipatory Grieving Related to Perceived Potential Loss of Personal Possessions

1. ANTICIPATORY GRIEVING RELATED TO PERCEIVED POTENTIAL LOSS OF SIGNIFICANT OTHER

190

Client Responses and/or Situations Needing Assessment

WELLNESS ORIENTED

Abortion
Crisis, of Family
Crisis, of Individual
Death, of Loved One
Divorce
Employment, Change in
Family Separation

Loss, of Loved One
Marital Status, Change in
Middle Age
Powerlessness
Relocation
Sleep Pattern Disturbance
Spiritual Distress

ILLNESS ORIENTED

Diagnosis, New
Illness, Chronic

Illness, Terminal

2. ANTICIPATORY GRIEVING RELATED TO PERCEIVED POTENTIAL LOSS OF PHYSIOPSYCHOSOCIAL WELL-BEING

Client Responses and/or Situations Needing Assessment

WELLNESS ORIENTED

Anorexia/Overeating
Divorce
Economic Status, Change in
Employment, Change in
Failure, Perceived
Financial Problems
Impotence
Insomnia
Loss, of Loved One

Loss, of Personal Items
Marital Status, Change in
Rape Trauma
Self-Esteem, Lowered
Social Status, Change in
Spiritual Distress
Weight Gain
Weight Loss

ILLNESS ORIENTED

Alcoholism
Amputation
Body Defacement
Diagnosis, New
Diagnostic Studies
Hospitalization
Hysterectomy

Mastectomy
Mental Illness, Suicide
  Ideation
Paralysis
Substance Abuse
Tubal Ligation
Vasectomy

3. ANTICIPATORY GRIEVING RELATED TO PERCEIVED POTENTIAL LOSS OF PERSONAL POSSESSIONS

Client Responses and/or Situations Needing Assessment

WELLNESS ORIENTED

Crisis, of Family
Crisis, of Individual
Death
Divorce
Economic Status, Change in
Employment, Change in
Financial Problems
Incarceration
Loss, of Loved One

Loss, of Personal Items
Marital Status, Change in
Powerlessness
Relocation
Retirement
Separation
Sleep Pattern Disturbance
Social Status, Change in

DIAGNOSTIC CATEGORY: GRIEVING, DYSFUNCTIONAL

†*Definition*: A condition in which the individual experiences delayed or exaggerated response to a perceived, actual, or potential loss.

Defining Characteristics

Verbal expression of distress at loss
Denial of loss
Expression of guilt
Expression of unresolved issues
Anger
Sadness
Crying
Difficulty in expressing loss
Alteration in eating habits
Alteration in sleep patterns
Alteration in dream patterns
Alteration in activity level
Alteration in libido
Idealization of lost object
Reliving of past experiences
Interference with life functioning
Developmental regression
Labile affect
Alterations in concentration and/or pursuits of tasks

Nursing Diagnoses Based on Identified Etiologies

Dysfunctional Grieving Related to Actual or Perceived Object Loss

Dysfunctional Grieving Related to Thwarted Grieving Response to Loss

Dysfunctional Grieving Related to Absence of Anticipatory Grieving

Dysfunctional Grieving Related to Chronic Fatal Illness

Dysfunctional Grieving Related to Loss of Significant Others

Dysfunctional Grieving Related to Loss of Physiopsychosocial Well-Being

Dysfunctional Grieving Related to Loss of Personal Possessions

1. DYSFUNCTIONAL GRIEVING RELATED TO ACTUAL OR PERCEIVED OBJECT LOSS

Comment: Object loss is used in the broadest sense to include people, possessions, a job, status, home, ideals, parts and processes of the body, etc.)

Client Responses and/or Situations Needing Assessment

WELLNESS ORIENTED

Abortion
Anorexia/Overeating
Crisis, of Individual
Death
Divorce
Economic Status, Change in
Employment, Change in
Failure, Perceived
Family Separation
Financial Problems
Impotence
Incarceration
Loss, of Loved One
Loss, of Personal Items
Marital Status, Change in
Powerlessness
Rape Trauma
Relocation
Retirement
Self-Esteem, Lowered
Separation
Sleep Pattern Disturbance
Social Status, Change in
Spiritual Distress
Weight Gain
Weight Loss

ILLNESS ORIENTED

Amputation
Body Defacement
Depression, Severe
Diagnosis, New

Diagnostic Studies
Hospitalization
Illness
Illness, Chronic
Illness, Terminal
Mastectomy

Mental Illness, Suicidal Ideation
Paralysis
Substance Abuse
Tubal Ligation
Vasectomy

2. DYSFUNCTIONAL GRIEVING RELATED TO THWARTED GRIEVING RESPONSE TO LOSS

Client Responses and/or Situations Needing Assessment

See Diagnostic Category: Grieving, Dysfunctional—Grieving Related to Actual or Perceived Object Loss

3. DYSFUNCTIONAL GRIEVING RELATED TO ABSENCE OF ANTICIPATORY GRIEVING

Client Responses and/or Situations Needing Assessment

See Diagnostic Category: Grieving, Dysfunctional—Grieving Related to Actual or Perceived Object Loss

4. DYSFUNCTIONAL GRIEVING RELATED TO CHRONIC FATAL ILLNESS

Client Responses and/or Situations Needing Assessment

WELLNESS ORIENTED

Abortion
Death, Impending

Loss, of Loved One

ILLNESS ORIENTED

Depression, Severe
Diagnosis, New
Illness, Chronic

Illness, Terminal
Mental Illness, Suicidal
   Ideation

5. DYSFUNCTIONAL GRIEVING RELATED TO LOSS OF SIGNIFICANT OTHERS

Client Responses and/or Situations Needing Assessment

WELLNESS ORIENTED

Abortion
Crisis, of Family
Crisis, of Individual
Death
Employment, Change in

Family Separation
Loss, of Loved One
Marital Status, Changes in
Relocation

ILLNESS ORIENTED

Depression, Severe
Diagnosis, New
Illness, Chronic

Illness, Terminal
Mental Illness, Suicidal
   Ideation

6. DYSFUNCTIONAL GRIEVING RELATED TO LOSS OF PHYSIOPSYCHOSOCIAL WELL-BEING

Client Responses and/or Situations Needing Assessment

WELLNESS ORIENTED

Anorexia/Overeating
Economic Status, Change in

Employment, Change in
Failure, Perceived

Financial Problems
Impotence
Insomnia
Loss, of Loved One
Loss, of Personal Items
Marital Status, Change in
Middle Age

Parenting, Role Change in
Rape Trauma
Self-Esteem, Lowered
Social Status, Change in
Weight Gain
Weight Loss

ILLNESS ORIENTED

Amputation
Body Defacement
Depression, Severe
Diagnosis, New
Diagnostic Studies
Hospitalization
Hysterectomy

Mastectomy
Mental Illness, Suicidal
  Ideation
Paralysis
Substance Abuse
Tubal Ligation
Vasectomy

7. DYSFUNCTIONAL GRIEVING RELATED TO LOSS OF PERSONAL POSSESSIONS

Client Responses and/or Situations Needing Assessment

WELLNESS ORIENTED

Crisis, of Family
Crisis, of Individual
Death
Economic Status, Change in
Employment, Change in
Financial Problems
Incarceration

Loss, of Loved One
Loss, of Personal Items
Marital Status, Change in
Relocation
Retirement
Social Status, Change in

ILLNESS ORIENTED

Depression, Severe
Mental Illness, Suicidal Ideation

DIAGNOSTIC CATEGORY:
**HEALTH MAINTENANCE,
ALTERATION IN**

Definition: Inability to identify, manage, and/or seek out help to maintain health.

Defining Characteristics

Demonstrated lack of knowledge regarding basic health practices

Demonstrated lack of adaptive behaviors to internal or external environmental changes

Reported or observed inability to take responsibility for meeting basic health practices in any or all functional pattern areas

History of lack of health-seeking behavior

Expressed interest in improving health behaviors

Reported or observed lack of equipment, financial and/or other resources

Reported or observed impairment of personal support system

Nursing Diagnoses Based on Identified Etiologies

Alteration in Health Maintenance Related to Lack of or Significant Alteration in Communication Skills

Alteration in Health Maintenance Related to Lack of Ability to Make Deliberate and Thoughtful Judgments

Alteration in Health Maintenance Related to Perceptual or Cognitive Impairment

Alteration in Health Maintenance Related to Complete or Partial Lack of Gross and/or Fine Motor Skills

Alteration in Health Maintenance Related to Ineffective
    Individual Coping; Dysfunctional Grieving
Alteration in Health Maintenance Related to Lack of Ma-
    terial Resources
Alteration in Health Maintenance Related to Unachieved
    Development Tasks
Alteration in Health Maintenance Related to Ineffective
    Family Coping: Disabling Spiritual Distress

1. ALTERATION IN HEALTH MAINTENANCE RELATED TO LACK OF OR SIGNIFICANT ALTERATION IN COMMUNICATION SKILLS

(*Explanation*: This includes written, verbal, and/or gestures.)

Client Responses and/or Situations Needing Assessment

WELLNESS ORIENTED

Adolescence
Anorexia/Overeating
Childhood
Deafness
Depression, Moderate
Economic Status, Change in
Failure, Perceived
Financial Problems
Infancy
Insomnia

Loss, of Loved One
Loss, of Personal Items
Marital Status, Change in
Muteness
Powerlessness
Self-Esteem, Lowered
Social Isolation
Social Status, Change in
Weight Gain
Weight Loss

ILLNESS ORIENTED

Anesthesia
Anorexia Nervosa

Bulimia
Confusion

Congenital Abnormalities
Emotional Disorders
Level of Consciousness,
  Comatose

Level of Consciousness,
  Decreased
Substance Abuse

2. ALTERATION IN HEALTH MAINTENANCE RELATED TO LACK OF ABILITY TO MAKE DELIBERATE AND THOUGHTFUL JUDGMENTS

Client Responses and/or Situations Needing Assessment

WELLNESS ORIENTED

Adolescence
Agedness
Childhood
Coping, Ineffective
Crisis, of Family

Crisis, of Individual
Grieving
Infancy
Mental Retardation
Stress / Distress

ILLNESS ORIENTED

Cerebral Vascular Problems
Delirium
Level of Consciousness,
  Lowered

Mental Illness
Neurological Disease
Substance Abuse

3. ALTERATION IN HEALTH MAINTENANCE RELATED TO PERCEPTUAL OR COGNITIVE IMPAIRMENT

Client Responses and/or Situations Needing Assessment

WELLNESS ORIENTED

Agedness

Childhood

200

Infancy
Knowledge Deficit
Mental Retardation

Noncompliance
Sensory Overload

ILLNESS ORIENTED

Emotional Disorders
Hallucinations
Illness, Acute
Mental Illness

Mental Problems
Organic Brain Syndrome
Substance Abuse

4. ALTERATION IN HEALTH MAINTENANCE RELATED TO COMPLETE OR PARTIAL LACK OF GROSS AND/OR FINE MOTOR SKILLS

Client Responses and/or Situations Needing Assessment

WELLNESS ORIENTED

Agedness
Childhood

Infancy

ILLNESS ORIENTED

Cardiovascular Disease
Mental Illness, Catatonic
Musculoskeletal Disease
Neurological Disease

Neuromuscular Disease
Pain
Paralysis

5. ALTERATION IN HEALTH MAINTENANCE RELATED TO INEFFECTIVE INDIVIDUAL COPING: DYSFUNCTIONAL GRIEVING

Client Responses and/or Situations Needing Assessment

WELLNESS ORIENTED

Abortion
Anorexia/Overeating
Divorce
Economic Status, Change in
Employment, Loss of
Failure, Perceived
Financial Loss
Financial Problems
Insomnia
Loss, of Loved one
Loss, of Personal Items

Marital Status, Change in
Middle Age
Self-Esteem, Lowered
Sleep Pattern Disturbance
Social Isolation
Social Status, Change in
Weight Gain
Weight Loss
Withdrawal
Young Adulthood

ILLNESS ORIENTED

Amputation
Body Defacement
Depression, Severe
Hysterectomy
Impotence
Mastectomy

Mental Illness, Suicidal
  Ideation
Paralysis
Substance Abuse
Tubal Ligation
Vasectomy

6. ALTERATION IN HEALTH MAINTENANCE RELATED TO LACK OF MATERIAL RESOURCES

Client Responses and/or Situations Needing Assessment

WELLNESS ORIENTED

Crisis, of Individual
Distant Family
Financial Problems

Incarceration
Knowledge Deficit
Loss, of Loved One

Relocation   Social Status, Change in
Separation

ILLNESS ORIENTED

Accidents   Hospitalization
Dialysis   Illness

7. ALTERATION IN HEALTH MAINTENANCE RELATED TO UNACHIEVED DEVELOPMENT TASKS

Client Responses and/or Situations Needing Assessment

WELLNESS ORIENTED

Adolescence   Incarceration
Agedness   Infertility
Childhood   Marital Status, Change in
Divorce   Retirement

ILLNESS ORIENTED

Illness, Chronic

8. ALTERATION IN HEALTH MAINTENANCE RELATED TO INEFFECTIVE FAMILY COPING: DISABLING SPIRITUAL DISEASE

Client Responses and/or Situations Needing Assessment

WELLNESS ORIENTED

Abortion   Crisis, of Individual
Anxiety   Despair

Divorce
Economic Status, Change in
Employment, Loss of
Failure, Perceived
Family Separation
Fear
Financial Problems
Guilt
Hostility
Impotence
Loss, of Loved One
Loss, of Personal Items
Marital Status, Change in
Relocation
Self-Esteem, Lowered
Separation
Social Status, Change in
Stress/Distress

ILLNESS ORIENTED

Body Defacement
Delusions
Disease Processes
Hospitalization, Long-Term
Illness, Terminal
Mastectomy
Paralysis
Substance Abuse

DIAGNOSTIC CATEGORY: HOME MAINTENANCE MANAGEMENT, IMPAIRED

Definition: The client is unable to independently maintain a safe, growth-promoting immediate environment.

Defining Characteristics

SUBJECTIVE	OBJECTIVE
†† Household members express difficulty in maintaining their home in a comfortable fashion	Disorderly surroundings
	†† Unwashed or unavailable cooking equipment, clothes, or linen
†† Household members request assistance with home maintenance	†† Accumulation of dirt, food wastes, or excrement
	Offensive odors

SUBJECTIVE	OBJECTIVE
†† Household members describe outstanding debts or financial crisis	Inappropriate household temperature
	†† Overtaxed family members, e.g., exhausted, anxious family members
	Lack of necessary equipment or aids
	Presence of vermin or rodents
	†† Repeated hygienic disorders, infestation, or infections

Nursing Diagnoses Based on Etiologies

Impaired Home Maintenance Management Related to Disease or Injury of Individual or Family Member

Impaired Home Maintenance Management Related to Insufficient Organization or Planning

Impaired Home Maintenance Management Related to Insufficient Finances

Impaired Home Maintenance Management Related to Unfamiliarity with Neighborhood Resources

Impaired Home Maintenance Management Related to Impaired Cognitive or Emotional Functioning

Impaired Home Maintenance Management Related to Lack of Knowledge

Impaired Home Maintenance Management Related to Lack of Role Modeling

Impaired Home Maintenance Management Related to Inadequate Support Systems

1. IMPAIRED HOME MAINTENANCE MANAGEMENT RELATED TO DISEASE OR INJURY OF INDIVIDUAL OR FAMILY MEMBER

Client Responses and/or Situations Needing Assessment

ILLNESS ORIENTED

Accident
Alcoholism
Cancer
Cardiopulmonary Disease
Cardiovascular Disease
Endocrine Disease
Hospitalization, Long-Term
Illness, Acute
Illness, Chronic

Illness, Terminal
Mental Illness
Metabolic Disease
Musculoskeletal Disease
Neurological Disease
Neuromuscular Disease
Respiratory Disease
Substance Abuse

2. IMPAIRED HOME MAINTENANCE MANAGEMENT RELATED TO INSUFFICIENT ORGANIZATION OR PLANNING

Client Responses and/or Situations Needing Assessment

WELLNESS ORIENTED

Crisis, of Family
Crisis, of Individual
Knowledge Deficit
Mental Retardation

Middle Age
Noncompliance
Young Adulthood

ILLNESS ORIENTED

Mental Illness

3. IMPAIRED HOME MAINTENANCE MANAGEMENT RELATED TO INSUFFICIENT FINANCES

Client Responses and/or Situations Needing Assessment

WELLNESS ORIENTED

Economic Status, Change in
Employment, Change in

Financial Problems
Social Status, Change in

ILLNESS ORIENTED

Dialysis
Hospitalization, Prolonged
Illness, Chronic

Illness, Terminal
Surgery, Experimental

4. IMPAIRED HOME MAINTENANCE MANAGEMENT RELATED TO UNFAMILIARITY WITH NEIGHBORHOOD RESOURCES

Client Responses and/or Situations Needing Assessment

WELLNESS ORIENTED

Divorce
Marital Status, Change in
Relocation

Retirement
Separation
Vacation

5. IMPAIRED HOME MAINTENANCE MANAGEMENT RELATED TO IMPAIRED COGNITIVE OR EMOTIONAL FUNCTIONING

Client Responses and/or Situations Needing Assessment

WELLNESS ORIENTED

Agedness
Crisis, of Family

Crisis, of Individual
Knowledge Deficit

Mental Retardation
Noncompliance

Sensory Overload
Stress/Distress

ILLNESS ORIENTED

Alcoholism
Emotional Disorders
Illness, Acute

Mental Illness
Substance Abuse

6. IMPAIRED HOME MAINTENANCE MANAGEMENT RELATED TO LACK OF KNOWLEDGE

Client Responses and/or Situations Needing Assessment

WELLNESS ORIENTED

Adolescence
Agedness
Anxiety
Childhood
Depression, Moderate
Incarceration
Infancy

Language, Barriers to
Language, Foreign
Mental Retardation
Newborn
Reading Skills, Insufficient
Stress/Distress

ILLNESS ORIENTED

Dialysis
Disability

Immobility
Paralysis

7. IMPAIRED HOME MAINTENANCE MANAGEMENT RELATED TO LACK OF ROLE MODELING

Client Responses and/or Situations Needing Assessment

WELLNESS ORIENTED

Crisis, of Family
Crisis, of Individual
Divorce
Employment, Change in
Employment, Loss of
Employment, New
Family Separation

Loss, of Loved One
Loss, of Role Model
Marital Status, Change in
Relocation
Retirement
Separation

8. IMPAIRED HOME MAINTENANCE MANAGEMENT RELATED TO INADEQUATE SUPPORT SYSTEMS

Client Responses and/or Situations Needing Assessment

WELLNESS ORIENTED

Coping, Ineffective Family
Crisis, of Family
Death
Distant Family
Divorce

Loss, of Loved One
Marital Status, Change in
Relocation
Separation
Social Isolation

ILLNESS ORIENTED

Hospitalization, Prolonged
Illness, Chronic

Illness, Terminal
Isolation

DIAGNOSTIC CATEGORY: INJURY: POTENTIAL FOR

†*Definition:* A condition in which the individual is at risk of physical injury.

Defining Characteristics

INTERNAL

Biochemical:
- Regulatory function:
  - Sensory dysfunction
  - Integrative dysfunction
  - Effector dysfunction
- Tissue hypoxia
- Malnutrition
- Immune–autoimmune
- Abnormal blood profile:
  - Leukocytosis/ leukopenia
  - Altered clotting factors
  - Thrombocytopenia
  - Sickle cell
  - Thalassemia
  - Decreased hemoglobin

Physical:
- Broken skin
- Altered mobility

Developmental:
- Age
  - Physiological
  - Psychosocial

Psychological:
- Affective
- Orientation

EXTERNAL

Biological:
- Immunization level of community
- Microorganism

Chemical:
- Pollutants
- Poisons

Drugs:
- Pharmaceutical agents
- Alcohol
- Caffeine
- Nicotine
- Preservatives
- Cosmetics and dyes
- Nutrients (vitamins, food types)

Physical:
- Design, structure, and arrangement of community, building, and/or equipment
- Mode of transport/ transportation
- Nosocomial agents

People–Provider:
- Nosocomial agent
- Staffing patterns
- Cognitive, affective, and psychomotor factors

Nursing Diagnoses Based on Identified Etiologies

Potential for Injury Related to Internal Factors, Host
Potential for Injury Related to External Environment

1. POTENTIAL FOR INJURY RELATED TO INTERNAL FACTORS, HOST

A. BIOLOGICAL

Client Responses and/or Situations Needing Assessment

ILLNESS ORIENTED

Blood Dyscrasias
Cardiopulmonary Disease
Cardiovascular Disease

Collagen Disease
Infections
Nutritional Deficiencies

B. CHEMICAL

Client Responses and/or Situations Needing Assessment

WELLNESS ORIENTED

Allergies
Medications

Skin Changes

ILLNESS ORIENTED

Alcoholism
Poison, Ingested

Substance Abuse

C. PHYSIOLOGIC

Client Responses and/or Situations Needing Assessment

WELLNESS/ILLNESS ORIENTED

Immobility

Skin Changes

D. PSYCHOLOGIC PERCEPTION

Client Responses and/or Situations Needing Assessment

WELLNESS ORIENTED

Agedness
Childhood
Infancy

Knowledge Deficit
Mental Retardation

ILLNESS ORIENTED

Alcoholism
Level of Consciousness,
  Comatose
Level of Consciousness,
  Decreased

Mental Illness
Substance Abuse

E. DEVELOPMENTAL

Client Responses and/or Situations Needing Assessment

WELLNESS ORIENTED

Adolescence
Agedness
Childhood

Infancy
Middle Age

2. POTENTIAL FOR INJURY RELATED TO EXTERNAL ENVIRONMENT

A. BIOLOGICAL

Client Responses and/or Situations Needing Assessment

WELLNESS ORIENTED

Accidents

Skin Changes

ILLNESS ORIENTED

Infections

Trauma

B. CHEMICAL

Client Responses and/or Situations Needing Assessment

WELLNESS ORIENTED

Allergies
Poison, Food
Pollution, Air

Pollution, Water
Weather

ILLNESS ORIENTED

Alcoholism

Substance Abuse

C. PHYSIOLOGIC

Client Responses and/or Situations Needing Assessment

WELLNESS ORIENTED

Exercise, Overexertion from

Knowledge Deficit

ILLNESS ORIENTED

Hospitalization
Immobilization

Safety Hazards

D. PSYCHOLOGIC

Client Responses and/or Situations Needing Assessment

WELLNESS ORIENTED

Crisis, of Family

Crisis, of Individual

E. PEOPLE-PROVIDER

Client Responses and/or Situations Needing Assessment

ILLNESS ORIENTED

Hospitalization   Illness, Long-Term

**DIAGNOSTIC CATEGORY:
INJURY: POTENTIAL FOR
SUBCATEGORY 1:
POISONING, POTENTIAL FOR**

Definition: The client has accentuated risk of accidental exposure to or ingestion of drugs or dangerous products in doses sufficient to cause poisoning.

Defining Characteristics

Internal (individual) factors
    Reduced vision
    Verbalization of occupational setting without adequate
        safeguards
    Lack of safety or drug education
    Lack of proper precautions
    Cognitive or emotional difficulties
    Insufficient finances
External (environmental) factors
    Large supplies of drugs in house
    Medicines stored in unlocked cabinets accessible to
        children or confused persons
    Dangerous products placed or stored within the
        reach of children or confused persons
    Availability of illicit drugs potentially contaminated
        by poisonous additives
    Flaking, peeling paint or plaster in presence of
        young children
    Chemical contamination of food and water
    Unprotected contact with heavy metals or chemicals

Paint, lacquer, etc. in poorly ventilated areas or
without effective protection
Presence of poisonous vegetation
Presence of atmospheric pollutants

DIAGNOSTIC CATEGORY: INJURY: POTENTIAL FOR SUBCATEGORY 2: SUFFOCATION, POTENTIAL FOR

Definition: The client has accentuated risk of accidental
suffocation (inadequate air available for inhalation).

Defining Characteristics

Internal (individual) factors
Reduced olfactory sensation
Reduced motor abilities
Lack of safety education
Lack of safety precautions
Cognitive or emotional difficulties
Disease or injury process
External (environmental) factors
Pillow placed in an infant's crib
Vehicle warming in closed garage
Children playing with plastic bags or inserting small
objects into their mouths or noses
Discarded or unused refrigerators or freezers without
removed doors
Children left unattended in bathtubs or pools
Household gas leaks
Smoking in bed
Use of fuel-burning heaters not vented to outside
Low-strung clothesline

Pacifier hung around infant's head
Eating of large mouthfuls of food
Propped bottle placed in an infant's crib

DIAGNOSTIC CATEGORY:
INJURY: POTENTIAL FOR
   SUBCATEGORY 3:
    TRAUMA, POTENTIAL FOR

Definition: The client has accentuated risk of accidental tissue injury, e.g., wound, burn, fracture.

Defining Characteristics

Internal (individual) factors
    Weakness
    Poor vision
    Balancing difficulties
    Reduced temperature and/or tactile sensation
    Reduced large- or small-muscle coordination
    Reduced hand-eye coordination
    Lack of safety education
    Lack of safety precautions
    Insufficient finances to purchase safety equipment or
       effect repairs
    Cognitive or emotional difficulties
    History of previous trauma
External (environmental) factors
    Slippery floors, e.g., wet or highly waxed
    Snow or ice on stairs, walkways
    Unanchored rugs
    Bathtub without hand grip or antislip equipment
    Use of unsteady ladder or chairs
    Entering unlighted rooms
    Unsturdy or absent stair rails

216

Unanchored electric wires
Litter or liquid spills on floors or stairways
High beds
Children playing without gates at top of stairs
Obstructed passageways
Unsafe window protection in homes with young
   children
Inappropriate call-for-aid mechanisms for bedresting
   client
Pot handles facing toward front of stove
Bathing in very hot water, e.g., unsupervised bathing
   of young children
Potential igniting of gas leaks
Delayed lighting of gas burner or oven
Experimenting with chemicals or gasoline
Unscreened fires or heaters
Wearing of plastic aprons or flowing clothing around
   open flame
Children playing with matches, candles, cigarettes
Inadequately stored combustibles or corrosives, e.g.,
   matches, oily rags, lye
Highly flammable children's toys or clothing
Overloaded fuse boxes
Contact with rapidly moving machinery, industrial
   belts, or pulleys
Sliding on coarse bed linen or struggling within bed
   restraints
Faulty electrical plugs, frayed wires, or defective
   appliances
Contact with acids or alkalis
Playing with fireworks or gunpowder
Contact with intense cold
Overexposure to sun, sun lamps, radiotherapy
Use of cracked dishware or glasses
Knives stored uncovered
Guns or ammunition stored unlocked

Large icicles hanging from roof
Exposure to dangerous machinery
Children playing with sharp-edged toys
High-crime neighborhood and vulnerable client
Driving a mechanically unsafe vehicle
Driving after partaking of alcoholic beverages or
   drugs
Driving at excessive speeds
Driving without necessary visual aids
Children riding in the front seat of car
Smoking in bed or near oxygen
Overloaded electrical outlets
Grease waste collected on stoves
Use of thin or worn pot holders or mitts
Unrestrained babies riding in car
Nonuse or misuse of seat restraints
Nonuse or misuse of necessary headgear for
   motorized cyclists or young children carried on
   adult bicycles
Unsafe road or road-crossing conditions
Play or work near vehicle pathways, e.g., driveways,
   lanes, railroad tracks

DIAGNOSTIC CATEGORY: KNOWLEDGE DEFICIT (SPECIFY)

Definition: Lack of specific information.

Defining Characteristics

Verbalization of the problem
Inaccurate follow-through of instruction
Inadequate performance of test
Inappropriate or exaggerated behaviors, e.g., hysterical,
   hostile, agitated, apathetic

Statement of misconception
Request for information

Nursing Diagnoses Based on Identified Etiologies

Knowledge Deficit Related to Lack of Exposure
Knowledge Deficit Related to Lack of Recall
Knowledge Deficit Related to Information Misinterpretation
Knowledge Deficit Related to Cognitive Limitation
Knowledge Deficit Related to Lack of Interest in Learning
Knowledge Deficit Related to Unfamiliarity with Information Resources
Knowledge Deficit Related to Client's Request for No Information

1. KNOWLEDGE DEFICIT RELATED TO LACK OF EXPOSURE

Client Responses and/or Situations Needing Assessment

WELLNESS ORIENTED

Sensory Deprivation   Social Isolation

ILLNESS ORIENTED

Diagnosis, New   Surgery
Illness, Acute   Tests/Treatments

2. KNOWLEDGE DEFICIT RELATED TO LACK OF RECALL

Client Responses and/or Situations Needing Assessment

WELLNESS ORIENTED

Agedness
Anxiety
Childhood

Crisis, of Family
Crisis, of Individual
Stress/Distress

ILLNESS ORIENTED

Alcoholism

Substance Abuse

3. KNOWLEDGE DEFICIT RELATED TO INFORMATION MISINTERPRETATION

Client Responses and/or Situations Needing Assessment

WELLNESS/ILLNESS ORIENTED

Communication
Diagnostic Procedures
Exercise, Overexertion
    from

Habits
Nutrition
Tests/Treatments

4. KNOWLEDGE DEFICIT RELATED TO COGNITIVE LIMITATION

Client Responses and/or Situations Needing Assessment

WELLNESS ORIENTED

Agedness
Childhood

Infancy
Mental Retardation

5. KNOWLEDGE DEFICIT RELATED TO LACK OF INTEREST IN LEARNING

Client Responses and/or Situations Needing Assessment

WELLNESS ORIENTED

Adolescence
Agedness
Anxiety
Middle Age

Noncompliance
Stress/Distress
Young Adulthood

ILLNESS ORIENTED

Alcoholism
Substance Abuse

6. KNOWLEDGE DEFICIT RELATED TO UNFAMILIARITY WITH INFORMATION RESOURCES

Client Responses and/or Situations Needing Assessment

WELLNESS ORIENTED

Adolescence
Divorce
Marital Status, Change in
Middle Age

Relocation
Retirement
Vacation
Young Adulthood

7. KNOWLEDGE DEFICIT RELATED TO CLIENT'S REQUEST FOR NO INFORMATION

Client Responses and/or Situations Needing Assessment

WELLNESS ORIENTED

Knowledge Deficit

DIAGNOSTIC CATEGORY:
MOBILITY, IMPAIRED PHYSICAL

†*Definition:* A condition in which the individual is unable to experience the full range of motion and movement.

Defining Characteristics

Inability to purposefully move within the physical environment, including bed mobility, transfer, and ambulation

Reluctance to attempt movement

Limited range of motion

Decreased muscle strength, control, and/or mass

Imposed restrictions of movement, including mechanical; medical protocol

Impaired coordination

Nursing Diagnoses Based on Identified Etiologies

Impaired Physical Mobility Related to Intolerance to Activity/Decreased Strength and Endurance

Impaired Physical Mobility Related to Pain/Discomfort

Impaired Physical Mobility Related to Perceptual/Cognitive Impairment

Impaired Physical Mobility Related to Neuromuscular Impairment

Impaired Physical Mobility Related to Musculoskeletal Impairment

Impaired Physical Mobility Related to Depression/Severe Anxiety

1. IMPAIRED PHYSICAL MOBILITY RELATED TO INTOLERANCE TO ACTIVITY/DECREASED STRENGTH AND ENDURANCE

Client Responses and/or Situations Needing Assessment

WELLNESS ORIENTED

Agedness
Allergies
Circulation, Decreased
Depression, Moderate

Fatigue
Obesity
Stress/Distress

ILLNESS ORIENTED

Bedrest, Prolonged
Chemotherapy
Coughing, Severe
Depression, Severe
Diabetes Mellitus
Diaphoresis
Diarrhea
Fever
Fluid and Electrolyte
   Imbalance

Hospitalization, Long-Term
Illness, Acute
Illness, Chronic
Illness, Terminal
Immobility
Metabolic Diseases
Nutritional Deficiencies
Postoperative Period
Radiation Therapy
Vomiting

2. IMPAIRED PHYSICAL MOBILITY RELATED TO PAIN/DISCOMFORT

Client Responses and/or Situations Needing Assessment

WELLNESS ORIENTED

Allergies
Diagnostic Studies
Headache

Muscle Strain
Pregnancy

ILLNESS ORIENTED

Burns
Cardiopulmonary Disease
Cardiovascular Disease
Musculoskeletal Disease
Neurological Disease

Renal Disease
Respiratory Disease
Surgery
Traction
Trauma

3. IMPAIRED PHYSICAL MOBILITY RELATED TO PERCEPTUAL/ COGNITIVE IMPAIRMENT

Client Responses and/or Situations Needing Assessment

WELLNESS ORIENTED

Agedness
Childhood
Crisis, of Family
Crisis, of Individual
Depression, Moderate
Infancy

Knowledge Deficit
Language, Barriers to
Language, Foreign
Mental Retardation
Stress/Distress

ILLNESS ORIENTED

Alcoholism
Illness, Acute

Mental Illness
Substance Abuse

4. IMPAIRED PHYSICAL MOBILITY RELATED TO NEUROMUSCULAR IMPAIRMENT

Client Responses and/or Situations Needing Assessment

WELLNESS ORIENTED

Agedness

Birth, Breech

Birth, Cesarean   Birth, Premature

ILLNESS ORIENTED

Anesthesia   Neurological Disease
Cerebral Palsy   Neuromuscular Disease
Cerebral Vascular Problems   Paralysis
Level of Consciousness,   Spinal Cord Injury
  Comatose   Spinal Cord Lesion
Level of Consciousness,
  Decreased

5. IMPAIRED PHYSICAL MOBILITY RELATED TO MUSCULOSKELETAL IMPAIRMENT

Client Responses and/or Situations Needing Assessment

WELLNESS ORIENTED

Agedness   Depression, Moderate
Birth, Premature   Obesity

ILLNESS ORIENTED

Amputation   Level of Consciousness,
Anesthesia   Decreased
Bedrest   Muscular Dystrophy
Cancer   Musculoskeletal Disease
Cast   Pain
Congenital Abnormalities   Paralysis
Disability   Substance Abuse
Hospitalization, Prolonged   Traction
Illness, Terminal   Trauma
Level of Consciousness,
  Comatose

6. IMPAIRED PHYSICAL MOBILITY RELATED TO DEPRESSION/ SEVERE ANXIETY

Client Responses and/or Situations Needing Assessment

See Diagnostic Category: Anxiety

WELLNESS ORIENTED

Anxiety Related to Unconscious Conflict About Essential Values/Goals of Life

Anxiety Related to Threat to Self-Concept

Anxiety Related to Threat of Death

Anxiety Related to Threat to or Change in Health Status

Anxiety Related to Threat to or Change in Socioeconomic Status

Anxiety Related to Threat to or Change in Role Functioning

Anxiety Related to Threat to or Change in Environment

Anxiety Related to Threat to or Change in Interaction Patterns

Anxiety Related to Situational/Maturational Crisis

Anxiety Related to Interpersonal Transmission/Contagion

Anxiety Related to Unmet Needs

Suggested code for functional level classification

  0 Completely independent

  1 Requires use of equipment or device

  2 Requires help from another person for assistance, supervision, or teaching

  3 Requires help from another person and equipment or device

  4 Is dependent, does not participate in activity

DIAGNOSTIC CATEGORY: NONCOMPLIANCE (SPECIFY)

Definition: Noncompliance is a person's informed decision not to adhere to a therapeutic recommendation.

Defining Characteristics

††Behavior indicative of failure to adhere by direct observation, statements by client or significant others
Objective tests (physiological measures, detection of markers)
Evidence of development of complications
Evidence of exacerbation of symptoms
Failure to keep appointments
Failure to progress

Nursing Diagnoses Based on Identified Etiologies

Noncompliance Related to Client Belief System
Noncompliance Related to Client and Provider Relationships

1. NONCOMPLIANCE RELATED TO CLIENT BELIEF SYSTEM

(*Explanation*: This includes health beliefs, cultural influences and spiritual values.)

Client Responses and/or Situations Needing Assessment

WELLNESS ORIENTED

Agedness   Anxiety

Crisis, of Family
Crisis, of Individual
Knowledge Deficit
Loss, Personal
Middle Age

Pregnancy
Self-Esteem, Lowered
Sexual Dysfunction
Stress/Distress
Young Adulthood

2. NONCOMPLIANCE RELATED TO CLIENT AND PROVIDER RELATIONSHIPS

Client Responses and/or Situations Needing Assessment

WELLNESS ORIENTED

Adolescence
Agedness
Anxiety
Blindness
Communication, Lack of

Deafness
Fear
Sensory Impairment
Stress/Distress

ILLNESS ORIENTED

Consultation, Physician
Paralysis

Relocation, to Another Agency
Relocation, Within Agency

DIAGNOSTIC CATEGORY: NUTRITION, ALTERATION IN: LESS THAN BODY REQUIREMENTS

†*Definition:* A condition in which the individual has inadequate intake of nutrients in relation to metabolic needs.

Defining Characteristics

Loss of weight with adequate food intake
20% or more under ideal body weight

Reported inadequate food intake less than RDA (Recommended Daily Allowance)

Weakness of muscles required for swallowing or mastication

Reported or evidence of lack of food

Lack of interest in food

Perceived inability to ingest food

Aversion to eating

Reported altered taste sensation

Satiety immediately after ingesting food

Abdominal pain with or without pathology

Sore, inflamed buccal cavity

Capillary fragility

Abdominal cramping

Diarrhea and/or steatorrhea

Hyperactive bowel sounds

Pale conjunctivae and mucous membranes

Poor muscle tone

Excessive loss of hair

Lack of information

Misconceptions

Nursing Diagnoses Based on Identified Etiologies

Alteration in Nutrition: Less Than Body Requirements Related to Inability to Ingest Foods

Alteration in Nutrition: Less Than Body Requirements Related to Inability to Digest Foods

Alteration in Nutrition: Less Than Body Requirements Related to Inability to Absorb Nutrients

1. ALTERATION IN NUTRITION: LESS THAN BODY REQUIREMENTS RELATED TO INABILITY TO INGEST FOODS

(*Explanation*: The causative factors may include biological, psychological, or economic factors.)

Client Responses and/or Situations Needing Assessment

WELLNESS ORIENTED

Adolescence
Anorexia/Overeating
Anxiety
Crisis, of Individual
Dental Problems
Dentures, Ill-Fitting
Diets, Fad
Economic Status, Change in
Employment, Change in
Financial Problems
Insomnia
Knowledge Deficit
Medications
Pregnancy
Social Isolation
Social Obligations
Stress/Distress

ILLNESS ORIENTED

Alcoholism
Anorexia Nervosa
Cancer
Chemotherapy
Congenital Abnormalities
Cough, Chronic
Dehydration
Fluid and Electrolyte
  Imbalance
Infant, Isolette
Infant, Premature
Infection
Infection, Throat
Malnutrition
Nausea
Nutrition, TPN
Nutritional Deficiencies
Nutritional Disease
Oral Disease
Pain
Paralysis
Parenteral Therapy
Radiation Therapy
Respiratory Disease
Substance Abuse
Surgery, Oral
Trauma, Face
Tumor
Vomiting
Vomiting, Projectile

2. ALTERATION IN NUTRITION: LESS THAN BODY REQUIREMENTS RELATED TO INABILITY TO DIGEST FOODS

(*Explanation*: The causative factors may include biological, psychological, or economic factors.)

Client Responses and/or Situations Needing Assessment

WELLNESS ORIENTED

Agedness
Allergies
Infant, Breastfeeding

Travel, Change in Food
Travel, Change in Water

ILLNESS ORIENTED

Alcoholism
Cancer
Celiac Disease
Congenital Abnormalities
Dehydration
Diarrhea
Endocrine Disease
Fluid and Electrolyte
   Imbalance

Gastroenteritis
Gastrointestinal Disease
Infant, Premature
Metabolic Disease
Parasites
Phenylketonuria (PKU)
Poisons
Substance Abuse

3. ALTERATION IN NUTRITION: LESS THAN BODY REQUIREMENTS RELATED TO INABILITY TO ABSORB NUTRIENTS

(*Explanation*: The causative factors may include biological, psychological, or economic factors.)

Potential Client Problems and/or Situations Needing Asssessment

ILLNESS ORIENTED

Alcoholism
Celiac Disease
Congenital Abnormalities
Cystic Fibrosis
Diabetes Mellitus
Diarrhea
Dehydration
Gastroenteritis
Gastrointestinal Disease
Intestinal Obstruction
Megacolon
Metabolic Disease
Parasites
Phenylketonuria (PKU)
Substance Abuse

DIAGNOSTIC CATEGORY: NUTRITION, ALTERATION IN: MORE THAN BODY REQUIREMENTS

†*Definition:* A condition in which the individual has more than adequate intake of nutrients in relation to metabolic needs.

Defining Characteristics

Weight 10% over ideal for height and frame
††Weight 20% over ideal for height and frame
††Triceps skin fold greater than 15 mm in men and 25 mm in women
Sedentary activity level

Reported or observed dysfunctional eating patterns
  Pairing food with other activities
  Concentrating food intake at end of day
  Eating in response to external cues, e.g., time of day,
    social situation
  Eating in response to internal cues other than hunger
    such as anxiety

Nursing Diagnoses Based on Identified Etiologies

Alteration in Nutrition: More Than Body Requirements
  Related to Excessive Intake in Relationship to Metabolic
  Need

1. ALTERATION IN NUTRITION: MORE THAN BODY REQUIREMENTS RELATED TO EXCESSIVE INTAKE IN RELATIONSHIP TO METABOLIC NEED

Client Responses and/or Situations Needing Assessment

WELLNESS ORIENTED

Adolescence	Knowledge Deficit
Agedness	Middle Age
Childhood	Obesity
Culture/Values	Pregnancy
Infancy	Sensory Deprivation

ILLNESS ORIENTED

Body Defacement	Cardiovascular Disease
Bulimia	Cerebral Vascular Problems

Emotional Disorders   Nutritional Disease

DIAGNOSTIC CATEGORY: NUTRITION, ALTERATION IN: POTENTIAL FOR MORE THAN BODY REQUIREMENTS

†*Definition:* A condition in which the individual has the potential for more than adequate intake of nutrients in relation to metabolic needs.

Defining Characteristics

†† Reported or observed obesity in one or both parents
†† Rapid transition across growth percentiles in infants or children
Reported use of solid food as major food source before 5 months of age
Observed use of food as reward or comfort measure
Reported or observed higher baseline weight at beginning of each pregnancy
Dysfunctional eating patterns
    Pairing food with other activities
    Concentrating food intake at end of day
    Eating in response to external cues, e.g., time of day, social situation
    Eating in response to internal cues other than hunger such as anxiety

Nursing Diagnoses Based on Identified Etiologies

Alteration in Nutrition: Potential for More Than Body Requirements Related to Hereditary Predisposition

Alteration in Nutrition: Potential for More Than Body Requirements Related To Excessive Energy Intake During Late Gestational Life, Early Infancy, and Adolescence

Alteration in Nutrition: Potential for More Than Body Requirements Related to Frequent, Close-Spaced Pregnancies

Alteration in Nutrition: Potential for More Than Body Requirements Related to Dysfunctional Psychological Conditioning in Relationship to Food

Alteration in Nutrition: Potential for More Than Body Requirements Related to Membership in Lower Socioeconomic Group

1. ALTERATION IN NUTRITION: POTENTIAL FOR MORE THAN BODY REQUIREMENTS RELATED TO HEREDITARY PREDISPOSITION

Client Responses and/or Situations Needing Assessment

See Diagnostic Category Alteration in Nutrition: More Than Body Requirements

WELLNESS ORIENTED

Hereditary Predisposition

2. ALTERATION IN NUTRITION: POTENTIAL FOR MORE THAN BODY REQUIREMENTS RELATED TO EXCESSIVE ENERGY INTAKE DURING LATE GESTATIONAL LIFE, EARLY INFANCY, AND ADOLESCENCE

Client Responses and/or Situations Needing Assessment

See Diagnostic Category Alteration in Nutrition: More Than Body Requirements

WELLNESS ORIENTED

Excessive energy intake during late gestational life, early infancy, and adolescence

3. ALTERATION IN NUTRITION: POTENTIAL FOR MORE THAN BODY REQUIREMENTS RELATED TO FREQUENT, CLOSE-SPACED PREGNANCIES

Client Responses and/or Situations Needing Assessment

See Diagnostic Category Alteration in Nutrition: More Than Body Requirements

WELLNESS ORIENTED

Frequent, close-spaced pregnancies

4. ALTERATION IN NUTRITION: POTENTIAL FOR MORE THAN BODY REQUIREMENTS RELATED TO DYSFUNCTIONAL PSYCHOLOGIC CONDITIONING IN RELATIONSHIP TO FOOD

Client Responses and/or Situations Needing Assessment

See Diagnostic Category Alteration in Nutrition: More Than Body Requirements

WELLNESS ORIENTED

Culture/Values	Habits
Depression, Moderate	Habits, Ethnic
Diet, Fad	Habits, Religious

ILLNESS ORIENTED

Anorexia Nervosa	
Bulimia	Mental Problems

5. ALTERATION IN NUTRITION: POTENTIAL FOR MORE THAN BODY REQUIREMENTS RELATED TO MEMBERSHIP IN LOWER SOCIOECONOMIC GROUP

Client Responses and/or Situations Needing Assessment

See Diagnostic Category Alteration in Nutrition: More Than Body Requirements

WELLNESS ORIENTED

Membership in lower socioeconomic group

DIAGNOSTIC CATEGORY: ORAL MUCOUS MEMBRANE, ALTERATION IN

†*Definition:* A condition in which the individual has an

alteration in the mucous membrane and/or structure of the mouth.

Defining Characteristics

Oral pain/discomfort
Coated tongue
Xerostomia (dry mouth)
Stomatitis
Oral lesions or ulcers
Lack of or decreased salivation
Leukoplakia
Edema

Hyperemia
Oral Plaque
Desquamation
Vesicles
Hemorrhagic gingivitis
Carious teeth
Halitosis

Nursing Diagnoses Based on Identified Etiologies

Alteration in Oral Mucous Membrane Related to Pathologic Condition—Oral Cavity

Alteration in Oral Mucous Membrane Related to Dehydration

Alteration in Oral Mucous Membrane Related to Trauma

Alteration in Oral Mucous Membrane Related to Nothing by Mouth (NPO) Instructions for More Than 24 Hours

Alteration in Oral Mucous Membrane Related to Ineffective Oral Hygiene

Alteration in Oral Mucous Membrane Related to Mouth Breathing

Alteration in Oral Mucous Membrane Related to Malnutrition

Alteration in Oral Mucous Membrane Related to Infection

Alteration in Oral Mucous Membrane Related to Lack of or Decreased Salivation

Alteration in Oral Mucous Membrane Related to Medication

1. ALTERATION IN ORAL MUCOUS MEMBRANE RELATED TO PATHOLOGIC CONDITION—ORAL CAVITY

Client Responses and/or Situations Needing Assessment

ILLNESS ORIENTED

Cancer
Dental Problems
Infection, Oral
Infection, Throat
Malnutrition

Nutritional Deficiencies
Nutritional Disease
Oral Disease
Radiation, Head/Neck

2. ALTERATION IN ORAL MUCOUS MEMBRANE RELATED TO DEHYDRATION

Client Responses and/or Situations Needing Assessment

ILLNESS ORIENTED

Burns
Diaphoresis
Diarrhea
Fever

Fluid and Electrolyte
  Imbalance
Renal Disease
Vomiting

3. ALTERATION IN ORAL MUCOUS MEMBRANE RELATED TO TRAUMA

A. CHEMICAL

Client Responses and/or Situations Needing Assessment

WELLNESS ORIENTED

Habit, Alcohol   Noxious Agents
Habit, Tobacco   Nutrition, Acid Foods

B. MECHANICAL

Client Responses and/or Situations Needing Assessment

WELLNESS ORIENTED

Dental Prosthesis   Dentures, Ill-Fitting

ILLNESS ORIENTED

Surgery, Oral   Tubes, Nasogastric
Tubes, Endotracheal

4. ALTERATION IN ORAL MUCOUS MEMBRANE RELATED TO NOTHING BY MOUTH (NPO) INSTRUCTIONS FOR MORE THAN 24 HOURS

Client Responses and/or Situations Needing Assessment

ILLNESS ORIENTED

Nothing by mouth (NPO) instructions for more than 24 hours

5. ALTERATION IN ORAL MUCOUS MEMBRANE RELATED TO INEFFECTIVE ORAL HYGIENE

Client Responses and/or Situations Needing Assessment

WELLNESS ORIENTED

Agedness
Childhood
Depression, Moderate

Infancy
Knowledge Deficit
Mental Retardation

ILLNESS ORIENTED

Alcoholism
Fracture, Jaw
Level of Consciousness,
    Comatose

Level of Consciousness,
    Lowered
Mental Retardation
Nothing by Mouth (NPO)
Substance Abuse

6. ALTERATION IN ORAL MUCOUS MEMBRANE RELATED TO MOUTH BREATHING

Client Responses and/or Situations Needing Assessment

WELLNESS ORIENTED

Birth, Premature
Deviated Septum

Infancy

ILLNESS ORIENTED

Blockage, Nasal
Cold
Level of Consciousness,
    Comatose
Level of Consciousness,
    Lowered

Oxygen Use
Pain
Sinusitis
Trauma, Nasal
Tubes, Nasogastric
Tumor, Nasal

7. ALTERATION IN ORAL MUCOUS MEMBRANE RELATED TO MALNUTRITION

Client Responses and/or Situations Needing Assessment

ILLNESS ORIENTED

Anorexia Nervosa
Celiac Disease
Endocrine Disease
Metabolic Disease

Nutrition, TPN
Nutritional Deficiency
Nutritional Disease

8. ALTERATION IN ORAL MUCOUS MEMBRANE RELATED TO INFECTION

Client Responses and/or Situations Needing Assessment

ILLNESS ORIENTED

Infection, Oral
Infection, Throat
Oral Diseases

Respiratory Disease
Sinusitis

9. ALTERATION IN ORAL MUCOUS MEMBRANE RELATED TO LACK OF OR DECREASED SALIVATION

Client Responses and/or Situations Needing Assessment

ILLNESS ORIENTED

Oral Disease
Parotitis
Ptyalism

10. ALTERATION IN ORAL MUCOUS MEMBRANE RELATED TO MEDICATION

Client Responses and/or Situations Needing Assessment

ILLNESS ORIENTED

Medication

DIAGNOSTIC CATEGORY: PARENTING, ALTERATION IN: ACTUAL OR POTENTIAL

Definition: Parenting is the ability of a nurturing figure(s) to create an environment that promotes the optimum growth and development of another human being. It is important to state as a preface to this diagnosis that adjustment to parenting in general is a normal maturational process that elicits nursing behaviors of prevention of potential problems and health promotion.

Defining Characteristics

ACTUAL AND POTENTIAL

Lack of parental attachment behaviors
    Inappropriate visual, tactile, auditory stimulation
    Negative identification of characteristics of infant/child
    Negative attachment of meanings to characteristics of infant/child
Constant verbalization of disappointment in gender or physical characteristics of infant/child
Verbalization of resentment toward infant/child
Verbalization of role inadequacy
†† Inattention to infant/child needs
    Verbal disgust of body functions of infant/child
    Noncompliance with health appointments for self and/or infant/child
†† Inappropriate caretaking behaviors (toilet training, sleep and rest, feeding)

Inappropriate or inconsistent discipline practices
Frequent accidents
Frequent illness
Growth and development lag in child
†† History of child abuse or abandonment by primary caretaker
Verbalizes desire to have child call parent by first name despite traditional cultural tendencies
Child receives care from multiple caretakers without consideration for the needs of the child
Compulsive seeking of role approval from others
ACTUAL
Abandonment
Runaway
Verbalization cannot control child
Evidence of physical and psychological trauma

Nursing Diagnoses Based on Identified Etiologies

(*Explanation*: These nursing diagnoses may be actual or potential; therefore, it must be specified which applies in order to clarify the diagnoses.)

(Specify) Alteration in Parenting Related to Lack of Available Role Model

(Specify) Alteration in Parenting Related to Ineffective Role Model

(Specify) Alteration in Parenting Related to Physical and Psychosocial Abuse of Nurturing Figure

(Specify) Alteration in Parenting Related to Lack of Support Between or From Significant Other(s)

(Specify) Alteration in Parenting Related to Unmet Social and Emotional Maturation Needs of Parenting Figures

(Specify) Alteration in Parenting Related to Interruption in Bonding Process

(Specify) Alteration in Parenting Related to Perceived Threat to Own Survival: Physical and Emotional

(Specify) Alteration in Parenting Related to Mental and/or Physical Illness

(Specify) Alteration in Parenting Related to Presence of Stress, Financial or Legal Problems, Recent Crisis, Cultural Move

(Specify) Alteration in Parenting Related to Lack of Knowledge

(Specify) Alteration in Parenting Related to Limited Cognitive Functioning

(Specify) Alteration in Parenting Related to Lack of Role Identity

(Specify) Alteration in Parenting Related to Lack of Appropriate Response of Child to Relationship

(Specify) Alteration in Parenting Related to Multiple Pregnancies

(Specify) Alteration in Parenting Related to Unrealistic Expectations for Self, Infant, Partner

1. (SPECIFY) ALTERATION IN PARENTING RELATED TO LACK OF AVAILABLE ROLE MODEL

Client Responses and/or Situations Needing Assessment

WELLNESS ORIENTED

Adolescence
Crisis, of Family
Crisis, of Individual
Divorce
Family, Single Parent

Incarceration
Marital Status, Change in
Parenting (Childrearing)
Separation
Sexual Dysfunction

ILLNESS ORIENTED

Alcoholism
Illness, Terminal
Mental Illness

Paralysis
Substance Abuse

2. (SPECIFY) ALTERATION IN PARENTING RELATED TO INEFFECTIVE ROLE MODEL

Client Responses and/or Situations Needing Assessment

WELLNESS ORIENTED

Abortion
Adolescence
Crisis, of Family
Crisis, of Individual

Divorce
Mental Retardation
Separation
Sexual Dysfunction

ILLNESS ORIENTED

Alcoholism
Illness, Terminal
Mental Illness

Paralysis
Substance Abuse

3. (SPECIFY) ALTERATION IN PARENTING RELATED TO PHYSICAL AND PSYCHOSOCIAL ABUSE OF NURTURING FIGURE

Client Responses and/or Situations Needing Assessment

WELLNESS ORIENTED

Abuse, Spouse

Family Violence

4. (SPECIFY) ALTERATION IN PARENTING RELATED TO LACK OF SUPPORT BETWEEN OR FROM SIGNIFICANT OTHER(S)

Client Responses and/or Situations Needing Assessment

WELLNESS ORIENTED

Abortion
Coping, Ineffective Family
Crisis, of Family
Death
Distant Family
Divorce

Fear
Loss, of Loved One
Relocation
Separation
Sexual Dysfunction

ILLNESS ORIENTED

Hospitalization, Prolonged
Illness, Chronic

Illness, Terminal
Isolation

5. (SPECIFY) ALTERATION IN PARENTING RELATED TO UNMET SOCIAL AND EMOTIONAL MATURATION NEEDS OF PARENTING FIGURES

Client Responses and/or Situations Needing Assessment

WELLNESS ORIENTED

Adolescence
Anorexia/Overeating
Divorce
Economic Status, Change in
Employment, Loss of
Failure, Perceived
Financial Loss
Financial Problems

Insomnia
Marital Status, Change in
Powerlessness
Self-Esteem, Lowered
Separation
Sexual Dysfunction
Social Status, Change in
Social Obligation

ILLNESS ORIENTED

Hospitalization   Illness, Chronic
Illness, Acute

6. (SPECIFY) ALTERATION IN PARENTING RELATED TO INTERRUPTION IN BONDING PROCESS

Client Responses and/or Situations Needing Assessment

WELLNESS ORIENTED

Anxiety   Crisis, of Individual
Birth, Premature   Relocation
Crisis, of Family   Stress/Distress

ILLNESS ORIENTED

Illness   Infant, Isolette
Illness, Acute   Paralysis

7. (SPECIFY) ALTERATION IN PARENTING RELATED TO PERCEIVED THREAT TO OWN SURVIVAL: PHYSICAL AND EMOTIONAL

Client Responses and/or Situations Needing Assessment

WELLNESS ORIENTED

Agedness   Diagnostic Studies
Anorexia/Overeating   Divorce

Economic Status, Change in
Employment, Loss of
Failure, Perceived
Financial Problems
Impotence
Insomnia
Loss, of Loved One
Loss, of Personal Items
Marital Status, Change in
Powerlessness
Self-Esteem, Lowered
Sexual Dysfunction
Social Isolation
Social Status, Change in
Spiritual Distress
Weight Gain
Weight Loss
Wellness, Change in
   Level of

ILLNESS ORIENTED

Alcoholism
Amputation
Body Defacement
Cardiovascular Disease,
   Severe
Diagnosis, New
Diagnostic Studies
Hysterectomy
Illness, Acute
Illness, Chronic
Illness, Sudden
Illness, Terminal
Mastectomy
Paralysis
Substance Abuse
Surgery, Impending
Tests/Treatments, Invasive
Tests/Treatments, Painful
Transplant Surgery,
   Impending
Tubal Ligation
Vasectomy

8. (SPECIFY) ALTERATION IN PARENTING RELATED TO MENTAL AND/OR PHYSICAL ILLNESS

Client Responses and/or Situations Needing Assessment

WELLNESS ORIENTED

Diagnostic Studies

Wellness, Change in Level of

ILLNESS ORIENTED

Diagnosis, New
Illness, Acute
Illness, Chronic

Illness, Sudden
Illness, Terminal

9. (SPECIFY) ALTERATION IN PARENTING RELATED TO PRESENCE OF STRESS, FINANCIAL OR LEGAL PROBLEMS, RECENT CRISIS, CULTURAL MOVE

Client Responses and/or Situations Needing Assessment

WELLNESS ORIENTED

Crisis, of Family
Crisis, of Individual
Divorce
Economic Status, Change in
Education
Employment, Change in
Financial Problems
Incarceration
Loss, of Loved One

Loss, of Personal Items
Marital Status, Change in
Marriage
Pregnancy
Relocation
Retirement
Separation
Social Status, Change in

ILLNESS ORIENTED

Disease Process

Illness

10. (SPECIFY) ALTERATION IN PARENTING RELATED TO LACK OF KNOWLEDGE

Client Responses and/or Situations Needing Assessment

250

WELLNESS ORIENTED

Knowledge Deficit Mental Retardation

ILLNESS ORIENTED

Mental Illness

11. (SPECIFY) ALTERATION IN PARENTING RELATED TO LIMITED COGNITIVE FUNCTIONING

Client Responses and/or Situations Needing Assessment

WELLNESS ORIENTED

Agedness   Knowledge Deficit
Childhood   Mental Retardation
Infancy   Noncompliance

ILLNESS ORIENTED

Alcoholism   Mental Illness
Illness, Acute   Substance Abuse

12. (SPECIFY) ALTERATION IN PARENTING RELATED TO LACK OF ROLE IDENTITY

Client Responses and/or Situations Needing Assessment

WELLNESS ORIENTED

Divorce   Marital Status, Change in
Family Addition   Separation
Family Crisis   Young Adulthood
Family Separation

13. (SPECIFY) ALTERATION IN PARENTING RELATED TO LACK OF APPROPRIATE RESPONSE OF CHILD TO RELATIONSHIP

Client Responses and/or Situations Needing Assessment

WELLNESS ORIENTED

Lack of appropriate response of child to relationship

14. (SPECIFY) ALTERATION IN PARENTING RELATED TO MULTIPLE PREGNANCIES

Client Responses and/or Situations Needing Assessment

WELLNESS ORIENTED

Pregnancies, Multiple

15. (SPECIFY) ALTERATION IN PARENTING RELATED TO UNREALISTIC EXPECTATIONS FOR SELF, INFANT, PARTNER

Client Responses and/or Situations Needing Assessment

WELLNESS ORIENTED

Adolescence
Anorexia/Overeating
Communication, Impaired
Depression, Moderate
Divorce
Fear
Marital Status, Change in
Separation
Social Isolation

DIAGNOSTIC CATEGORY: POWERLESSNESS

Definition: The perception of the individual that one's own action will not significantly affect an outcome. Powerlessness is the perceived lack of control over a current situation or immediate happening.

Defining Characteristics

SEVERE

Verbal expressions of having no control or influence over situation

Verbal expressions of having no control or influence over outcome

Verbal expressions of having no control over self-care

Depression over physical deterioration that occurs despite patient compliance with regimens

Apathy

MODERATE

Nonparticipation in care or decision making when opportunities are provided

Expressions of dissatisfaction and frustration over inability to perform previous tasks and/or activities

Does not monitor progress

Expression of doubt regarding role performances

Reluctance to express true feelings, fearing alienation from care givers

Inability to seek information regarding care

Dependence on others that may result in irritability, resentment, anger, and guilt

Does not defend self-care practices when challenged
Passivity

LOW

Passivity
Expressions of uncertainty about fluctuating energy levels

Nursing Diagnoses Based on Identified Etiologies

Powerlessness Related to Health Care Environment
Powerlessness Related to Interpersonal Interaction
Powerlessness Related to Illness-Related Regimen
Powerlessness Related to Life Style of Helplessness

1. POWERLESSNESS RELATED TO HEALTH CARE ENVIRONMENT

Client Responses and/or Situations Needing Assessment

ILLNESS ORIENTED

Diagnostic Studies	Illness
Hospitalization	Relocation

2. POWERLESSNESS RELATED TO INTERPERSONAL INTERACTION

Client Responses and/or Situations Needing Assessment

WELLNESS ORIENTED

Abuse	Anxiety
Adolescence	Childhood
Agedness	Communication, Lack of

Coping, Ineffective Family
Coping, Ineffective Individual
Crisis, of Family
Crisis, of Individual
Culture/Values
Divorce
Economic Status, Change in
Education, Change in
Failure, Perceived
Fear
Financial Loss
Financial Problems
Infancy
Insomnia
Knowledge Deficit
Life Style, Change in
Loss, of Loved One
Loss, of Personal Items
Marriage, New
Middle Age
Pregnancy
Relocation
Retirement
Self-Esteem, Disturbance in
Separation
Sexual Dysfunction
Social Isolation
Social Obligation
Social Status, Change in
Stress/Distress
Young Adulthood

ILLNESS ORIENTED

Accidents
Hospitalization

Illness
Pain

3. POWERLESSNESS RELATED TO ILLNESS-RELATED REGIMEN

Client Responses and/or Situations Needing Assessment

ILLNESS ORIENTED

Accidents
Diagnosis, New
Diagnostic Studies
Dialysis
Hospitalization
Illness, Acute
Illness, Chronic
Illness, Sudden
Illness, Terminal
Pain
Paralysis
Surgery, Impending
Tests/Treatments, Invasive
Tests/Treatments, Painful
Transplant Surgery, Impendir

4. POWERLESSNESS RELATED TO LIFE STYLE OF HELPLESSNESS

Client Responses and/or Situations Needing Assessment

WELLNESS ORIENTED

Life Style, Helplessness
Life Style, Nonassertive

DIAGNOSTIC CATEGORY: RAPE TRAUMA SYNDROME

Definition: Rape is forced and violent sexual penetration against the victim's will and without the victim's consent. The trauma syndrome that develops from an attack or attempted attack includes an acute phase of disorganization of the victim's life style and a long-time process of reorganization of life style. This syndrome includes the following three subcomponents: A, B, and C.

A. RAPE TRAUMA

Defining Characteristics

Acute Phase
    Emotional Reactions
        Anger
        Embarrassment
        Fear of physical violence and death
        Humiliation
        Revenge
        Self-blame
    Multiple Physical Symptoms
        Gastrointestinal irritability
        Genitourinary discomfort
        Muscle tension

Sleep pattern disturbance
Long-Term Phase
Changes in Life Style
Changes in residence
Dealing with repetitive nightmares and phobias
Seeking family support
Seeking social network support

B. COMPOUND REACTION

Defining Characteristics

All defining characteristics listed under rape trauma
Reactivated symptoms of such previous conditions, i.e.,
physical illness, psychiatric illness
Reliance on alcohol and/or drugs

C. SILENT REACTION

Defining Characteristics

Abrupt changes in relationships with men
Increase in nightmares
Increasing anxiety during interview, i.e., blocking of as-
sociations, long periods of silence, minor stuttering, phys-
ical distress
Marked changes in sexual behavior
No verbalization of the occurrence of rape
Sudden onset of phobic reactions

DIAGNOSTIC CATEGORY:
SELF-CARE DEFICIT:
FEEDING, BATHING/HYGIENE,
DRESSING/GROOMING, TOILETING

†*Definition:* A condition in which the individual is unable
to provide self-care in one or all of the following areas:

feeding, bathing/hygiene, dressing/grooming, and toileting.

A. SELF-FEEDING DEFICIT
(LEVEL 0 to 4)+

Defining Characteristics

Inability to bring food from a receptacle to the mouth

B. SELF-BATHING/HYGIENE DEFICIT
(LEVEL 0 to 4)+

Defining Characteristics

††Inability to wash body or body parts
 Inability to obtain or get to water source
 Inability to regulate temperature or flow

C. SELF-DRESSING/GROOMING DEFICIT
 (LEVEL 0 to 4)+

Defining Characteristics

††Impaired ability to put on or take off necessary items
  of clothing
 Impaired ability to obtain or replace articles of clothing
 Impaired ability to fasten clothing
 Inability to maintain appearance to satisfactory level

D. SELF-TOILETING DEFICIT
 (LEVEL 0 to 4)+

Defining Characteristics

††Unable to get to toilet or commode
††Unable to sit on or rise from toilet or commode
††Unable to manipulate clothing for toileting
††Unable to carry out proper toilet hygiene
 Unable to flush toilet or empty commode
 For definition of code see Mobility, Impaired Physical
  (p. 225)

Nursing Diagnoses Based on Identified Etiologies

(*Explanation*: These diagnoses may be specified to include visual, auditory, kinesthetic, gustatory, tactile, or olfactory perceptions.)

Self-Care Deficit (Specify) Related to Intolerance to Activity, Decreased Strength and Endurance

Self-Care Deficit (Specify) Related to Pain, Discomfort

Self-Care Deficit (Specify) Related to Perceptual or Cognitive Impairment

Self-Care Deficit (Specify) Related to Neuromuscular Impairment

Self-Care Deficit (Specify) Related to Musculoskeletal Impairment

Self-Care Deficit (Specify) Related to Depression, Severe Anxiety

Self-Care Deficit: Toileting Related to Impaired Transfer Ability

Self-Care Deficit: Toileting Related to Impaired Mobility Status

1. SELF-CARE DEFICIT (SPECIFY) RELATED TO INTOLERANCE TO ACTIVITY, DECREASED STRENGTH AND ENDURANCE

Client Responses and/or Situations Needing Assessment

WELLNESS ORIENTED

Accidents	Altitude, Low
Agedness	Anxiety
Allergies	Cough
Altitude, High	Crisis, of Family

Crisis, of Individual
Depression, Moderate
Diet, Starvation
Exercise, Overexertion from

Fatigue
Insomnia
Obesity
Stress/Distress

ILLNESS ORIENTED

Bedrest, Prolonged
Cardiopulmonary Disease
Cardiovascular Disease
Chemotherapy
Cough, Chronic
Cough, Severe
Depression, Severe
Diabetes Mellitus
Diaphoresis
Diarrhea
Endocrine Disease
Fever
Fluid and Electrolyte
  Imbalance

Hospitalization,
  Long-Term
Illness, Chronic
Illness, Terminal
Immobility
Immunological Disease
Metabolic Disease
Musculoskeletal Disease
Neurological Disease
Nutritional Deficiencies
Pain
Radiation Therapy
Respiratory Disease
Vomiting/Diarrhea

2. SELF-CARE DEFICIT (SPECIFY) RELATED TO PAIN, DISCOMFORT

Client Responses and/or Situations Needing Assessment

Allergies
Diagnostic Studies
Headache

Muscle Strain
Poison
Pregnancy

ILLNESS ORIENTED

Burns
Cardiopulmonary Disease

Injury, Back
Injury, Neck

Respiratory Disease
Surgery, Abdominal

Surgery, Chest
Trauma

3. SELF-CARE DEFICIT (SPECIFY) RELATED TO PERCEPTUAL OR COGNITIVE IMPAIRMENT

Client Responses and/or Situations Needing Assessment

WELLNESS ORIENTED

Agedness
Childhood
Crisis, of Family
Crisis, of Individual
Depression, Moderate
Infancy

Knowledge, Deficit
Language, Barriers to
Language, Foreign
Mental Retardation
Motivation
Noncompliance

ILLNESS ORIENTED

Alcoholism
Emotional Disorders
Hallucination
Illness, Acute
Level of Consciousness, Comatose

Level of Consciousness, Decreased
Mental Problems
Organic Brain Syndrome
Substance Abuse

4. SELF-CARE DEFICIT (SPECIFY) RELATED TO NEUROMUSCULAR IMPAIRMENT

Client Responses and/or Situations Needing Assessment

WELLNESS ORIENTED

Agedness

Birth, Breech

Birth, Cesarean
Birth, Premature

ILLNESS ORIENTED

Anesthesia
Cerebral Palsy
Cerebral Vascular Problems
Level of Consciousness,
  Comatose
Level of Consciousness,
  Decreased

Neurological Disease
Neuromuscular Disease
Paralysis
Spinal Cord Injury

5. SELF-CARE DEFICIT (SPECIFY) RELATED TO MUSCULOSKELETAL IMPAIRMENT

Client Responses and/or Situations Needing Assessment

WELLNESS ORIENTED

Agedness
Birth, Premature
Depression

Disability
Obesity

ILLNESS ORIENTED

Amputation
Anesthesia
Bedrest
Cancer
Cast
Congenital Abnormalities
Disability
Hospitalization, Prolonged
Illness, Terminal
Level of Consciousness,
  Comatose

Level of Consciousness,
  Decreased
Muscular Dystrophy
Musculoskeletal Disease
Pain
Paralysis
Substance Abuse
Traction
Trauma

6. SELF-CARE DEFICIT (SPECIFY) RELATED TO DEPRESSION, SEVERE ANXIETY

Client Responses and/or Situations Needing Assessment

WELLNESS ORIENTED

Anxiety Related to Unconscious Conflict About Essential Values/Goals of Life

Anxiety Related to Threat to Self-Concept

Anxiety Related to Threat of Death

Anxiety Related to Threat to or Change in Health Status

Anxiety Related to Threat to or Change in Socioeconomic Status

Anxiety Related to Threat to or Change in Role Functioning

Anxiety Related to Threat to or Change in Environment

Anxiety Related to Threat to or Change in Interaction Patterns

Anxiety Related to Situational/Maturational Crisis

Anxiety Related to Interpersonal Transmission/Contagion

Anxiety Related to Unmet Needs

7. SELF-CARE DEFICIT: TOILETING RELATED TO IMPAIRED TRANSFER ABILITY

Client Responses and/or Situations Needing Assessment

WELLNESS ORIENTED

Agedness   Mental Retardation

ILLNESS ORIENTED

Cerebral Palsy
Disability
Mental Illness, Catatonia
Muscular Dystrophy
Musculoskeletal Disease

Neurological Disease
Neuromuscular Disease
Paralysis
Spinal Cord Injury
Spinal Cord Lesion

8. SELF-CARE DEFICIT: TOILETING RELATED TO IMPAIRED MOBILITY STATUS

Client Responses and/or Situations Needing Assessment

WELLNESS ORIENTED

Agedness

Mental Retardation

ILLNESS ORIENTED

Cerebral Palsy
Disability
Level of Consciousness,
    Comatose
Level of Consciousness,
    Decreased
Mental Illness, Catatonia
Mental Problems

Muscular Dystrophy
Musculoskeletal Disease
Neurological Disease
Neuromuscular Disease
Paralysis
Spinal Cord Injury
Spinal Cord Lesion

DIAGNOSTIC CATEGORY: SELF-CONCEPT, DISTURBANCE IN: BODY IMAGE, SELF-ESTEEM, ROLE PERFORMANCE, PERSONAL IDENTITY

Definition: A disturbance in self-concept is a disruption in the way one perceives one's body image, self-esteem, role performance, and/or personal identity. (These four sub-components in turn have their own etiologies and defining characteristics.)

A. BODY IMAGE, DISTURBANCE IN

Defining Characteristics

Verbal response to actual or perceived change in structure and/or function

Nonverbal response to actual or perceived change in structure and/or function

Nursing Diagnoses Based on Etiologies

Disturbance in Body Image Related to Biophysical

Disturbance in Body Image Related to Cognitive Perceptual

Disturbance in Body Image Related to Psychosocial

Disturbance in Body Image Related to Cultural or Spiritual

1. DISTURBANCE IN BODY IMAGE RELATED TO BIOPHYSICAL

Client Responses and/or Situations Needing Assessment

WELLNESS ORIENTED

Abortion	Obesity
Adolescence	Rape Trauma
Anorexia/Overeating	Skin Changes
Impotence	Weight Gain
Insomnia	Weight Loss

ILLNESS ORIENTED

Amputation	Arthritis
Anorexia Nervosa	Body Defacement

Bulimia
Hysterectomy
Immobility
Mastectomy
Paralysis

Surgery
Trauma
Tubal Ligation
Vasectomy

2. DISTURBANCE IN BODY IMAGE RELATED TO COGNITIVE PERCEPTUAL

Client Responses and/or Situations Needing Assessment

WELLNESS ORIENTED

Adolescence
Agedness
Childhood
Coping, Individual
Crisis, of Family
Crisis, of Individual
Depression, Moderate

Diagnostic Studies
Fear
Grieving
Infancy
Mental Retardation
Middle Age
Young Adulthood

ILLNESS ORIENTED

Cerebral Vascular Problems
Delirium
Depression, Severe
Diagnosis, New
Diagnostic Studies
Emotional Disorders

Illness, Acute
Mental Illness
Mental Problems
Organic Brain Syndrome
Substance Abuse

3. DISTURBANCE IN BODY IMAGE RELATED TO PSYCHOSOCIAL

Client Responses and/or Situations Needing Assessment

WELLNESS ORIENTED

Adolescence
Agedness
Anorexia/Overeating
Anxiety
Child Abuse/Neglect
Crisis, of Family
Crisis, of Individual
Culture/Values
Economic Status,
    Change in
Employment, Change in
Failure, Perceived
Family Separation
Fear
Financial Problems
Impotence

Incarceration
Insomnia
Loss, of Loved One
Loss, of Personal Items
Marital Status, Change in
Obesity
Parenting (childrearing)
Pregnancy
Relocation
Retirement
Self-Concept, Lowered
Sexual Dysfunction
Social Isolation
Social Status, Change in
Weight, Gain
Weight, Loss

ILLNESS ORIENTED

Diagnosis, New
Diagnostic Studies
Emotional Disorders
Hospitalization

Illness, Acute
Illness, Chronic
Illness, Terminal
Substance Abuse

4. DISTURBANCE IN BODY IMAGE RELATED TO CULTURAL OR SPIRITUAL

Client Responses and/or Situations Needing Assessment

WELLNESS ORIENTED

Anxiety
Birth, Premature
Fear

Self-Esteem, Lowered
Stress/Distress

ILLNESS ORIENTED

Delusions
Emotional Disorders
Hospitalization

Illness, Chronic
Illness, Terminal
Mental Illness

B. SELF-ESTEEM, DISTURBANCE IN

Defining Characteristics

Inability to accept positive reinforcement
Lack of follow-through
Nonparticipation in therapy
Not taking responsibility for self-care (self-neglect)
Self-destructive behavior
Lack of eye contact

Nursing Diagnoses Based on Etiologies

Disturbance in Self-Esteem Related to (Specify)

1. DISTURBANCE IN SELF-ESTEEM RELATED TO (SPECIFY)

††Client Responses and/or Situations Needing Assessment

††See Subcomponent: Body Image, Disturbance in

C. ROLE PERFORMANCE, DISTURBANCE IN

Defining Characteristics

Change in self-perception of role
Denial of role
Change in others' perception of role
Conflict in roles
Change in physical capacity to resume role
Lack of knowledge of role
Change in usual patterns of responsibility

268

Nursing Diagnoses Based on Identified Etiologies

Disturbance in Role Performance Related to (Specify)

1. DISTURBANCE IN ROLE PERFORMANCE RELATED TO (SPECIFY)

††Client Responses and/or Situations Needing Assessment

††See Subcomponent: Body Image, Disturbance in

D. PERSONAL IDENTITY, DISTURBANCE IN

Definition: Inability to distinguish between self and nonself

Defining Characteristics

To be developed

Nursing Diagnoses Based on Identified Etiologies

Disturbance in Personal Identity Related to (Specify)

1. DISTURBANCE IN PERSONAL IDENTITY RELATED TO (SPECIFY)

††Client Responses and/or Situations Needing Assessment

††See Subcomponent: Body Image, Disturbance in

DIAGNOSTIC CATEGORY:
SENSORY-PERCEPTUAL ALTERATION:
VISUAL, AUDITORY, KINESTHETIC,
GUSTATORY, TACTILE, OLFACTORY

†*Definition:* A condition in which the individual experiences
a change in therapeutic and/or social stimuli.

Defining Characteristics

Disoriented in time, in place, or with persons
Altered abstraction
Altered conceptualization
Change in problem-solving abilities
Reported or measured change in sensory acuity
Change in behavior pattern
Anxiety
Apathy
Change in usual response to stimuli
Indication of body-image alteration
Restlessness
Irritability
Altered communication patterns
Disorientation
Lack of concentration
Daydreaming
Hallucinations
Noncompliance
Fear
Depression
Rapid mood swings
Anger
Exaggerated emotional responses
Poor concentration

Disordered thought sequencing
Bizarre thinking
Visual and auditory distortions
Motor incoordination
Complaints of fatigue
Alteration in posture
Change in muscular tension
Inappropriate responses
Hallucinations

Nursing Diagnoses Based on Etiologies

(*Explanation*: These diagnoses may be specified to include visual, auditory, kinesthetic, gustatory, tactile, or olfactory perceptions.)

Sensory-Perceptual Alteration: (Specify) Related to Environmental Factors
Sensory-Perceptual Alteration: (Specify) Related to Altered Sensory Reception, Transmission, and/or Integration
Sensory-Perceptual Alteration: (Specify) Related to Chemical Alteration
Sensory-Perceptual Alteration: (Specify) Related to Psychologic Stress

1. SENSORY-PERCEPTUAL ALTERATION: (SPECIFY) RELATED TO ENVIRONMENTAL FACTORS

Explanation: This includes therapeutically and socially restricted environments.

Client Responses and/or Situations Needing Assessment

WELLNESS ORIENTED

Agedness   Disability

Grieving
Incarceration
Infant, Incubator

Mental Retardation
Relocation
Social Isolation

ILLNESS ORIENTED

Anesthesia
Bedrest
Hospitalization
Illness, Chronic
Illness, Sudden
Illness, Terminal
Intensive Care Units

Isolation, Hospital
Mental Illness
Paralysis
Surgery
Tests/Treatments, Painful
Traction

2. SENSORY-PERCEPTUAL ALTERATION: (SPECIFY) RELATED TO ALTERED SENSORY RECEPTION, TRANSMISSION, AND/OR INTEGRATION

Client Responses and/or Situations Needing Assessment

WELLNESS ORIENTED

Ankyloglossia
Birth
Blindness
Crisis, of Family
Crisis, of Individual
Dental Problems
Hearing Loss
Knowledge, Lack of
  Comprehension

Language, Barriers of
Language, Foreign
Language, Nonverbal
Mental Retardation
Skin Changes
Speech Impediment

ILLNESS ORIENTED

Alcoholism

Brain Tumor

Cardiovascular Disease
Cerebral Vascular Problems
CNS Depression
Congenital Abnormalities
Embolus
Infections, Ear
Intubation
Neurological Disease
Spinal Cord Injury

Substance Abuse
Surgery, Oral
Tracheostomy
Trauma
Trauma, Face
Trauma, Head
Trauma, Neck
Trauma, Oral

3. SENSORY-PERCEPTUAL ALTERATION: (SPECIFY) RELATED TO CHEMICAL ALTERATION

Explanation: This diagnosis includes endogenous and exogenous etiologies.

Client Responses and/or Situations Needing Assessment

WELLNESS ORIENTED

Allergies
Chemical
Hyperventilation
Medications, CNS
  Depressants

Medications, CNS
  Stimulants
Poison, Food
Pollution, Air
Pollution, Water

ILLNESS ORIENTED

Alcoholism
Ammonia, Elevated
BUN, Elevated
Fluid and Electrolyte
  Imbalance

Hypoxia
Poison, Ingested
Substance Abuse

4. SENSORY-PERCEPTUAL ALTERATION: (SPECIFY) RELATED TO PSYCHOLOGIC STRESS

Client Responses and/or Situations Needing Assessment

WELLNESS ORIENTED

Agedness
Anxiety
Crisis, of Family
Crisis, of Individual
Depression, Moderate

Fear
Knowledge Deficit
Lack of Stimuli
Perception, Inaccurate

ILLNESS ORIENTED

Alcoholism
Depression, Severe
Level of Consciousness,
  Comatose

Level of Consciousness,
  Decreased
Mental Illness
Mental Problems

DIAGNOSTIC CATEGORY: SEXUAL DYSFUNCTION

†*Definition:* A condition in which the individual experiences a biological-psychological-social alteration in sexuality.

Defining Characteristics

Verbalization of problem
Alterations in achieving perceived sex role
Actual or perceived limitation imposed by disease and/or therapy
Conflicts involving values
Alterations in achieving sexual satisfaction

Inability to achieve desired satisfaction
Seeking of confirmation of desirability
Alteration in relationship with significant other
Change in interest in self and others

Nursing Diagnoses Based on Identified Etiologies

Sexual Dysfunction Related to Ineffectual or Absent Role
  Models
Sexual Dysfunction Related to Physical Abuse
Sexual Dysfunction Related to Psychosocial Abuse
Sexual Dysfunction Related to Vulnerability
Sexual Dysfunction Related to Misinformation or Lack of
  Knowledge
Sexual Dysfunction Related to Values Conflict
Sexual Dysfunction Related to Lack of Privacy
Sexual Dysfunction Related to Lack of Significant Other
Sexual Dysfunction Related to Altered Body Structure or
  Function

1. SEXUAL DYSFUNCTION RELATED TO INEFFECTUAL OR ABSENT ROLE MODELS

Client Responses and/or Situations Needing Assessment

WELLNESS ORIENTED

Adolescence
Child Abuse/Neglect
Crisis, of Family
Crisis, of Individual
Divorce
Family, Single Parent
Incarceration
Young Adulthood

ILLNESS ORIENTED

Alcoholism
Emotional Disorders

Illness, Terminal   Paralysis
Mental Illness   Substance Abuse

2. SEXUAL DYSFUNCTION RELATED TO PHYSICAL ABUSE

Client Responses and/or Situations Needing Assessment

WELLNESS ORIENTED

Abuse, Sexual   Family Violence
Abuse, Spouse   Rape Trauma

ILLNESS ORIENTED

Hospitalization   Trauma, Unexplained
Impotence

3. SEXUAL DYSFUNCTION RELATED TO PSYCHOSOCIAL ABUSE

Client Responses and/or Situations Needing Assessment

WELLNESS ORIENTED

Abuse, Spouse   Incarceration
Crisis, Family   Marital Status, Change in
Divorce   Separation
Impotence

ILLNESS ORIENTED

Emotional Disorder   Mental Illness
Hospitalization

4. SEXUAL DYSFUNCTION RELATED TO VULNERABILITY

Client Responses and/or Situations Needing Assessment

WELLNESS ORIENTED

Anorexia

Child Abuse/Neglect

Culture/Values

Divorce

Economic Status, Change in

Failure, Perceived

Financial Problems

Impotence

Insomnia

Loss, of Loved One

Loss, of Personal Items

Marital Status, Change in

Middle Age

Powerlessness

Rape Trauma

Self-Esteem, Lowered

Separation

Social Status, Change in

Weight Gain

Weight Loss

ILLNESS ORIENTED

Alcoholism

Anorexia Nervosa

Bulimia

Emotional Disorders

Mental Illness

Paralysis

5. SEXUAL DYSFUNCTION RELATED TO MISINFORMATION OR LACK OF KNOWLEDGE

Client Responses and/or Situations Needing Assessment

WELLNESS ORIENTED

Adolescence

Agedness

Anxiety

Crisis, of Family

Crisis, of Individual

Impotence

Stress/Distress

Young Adulthood

ILLNESS ORIENTED

Cardiopulmonary Disease

Emotional Disorders

Endocrine Disease
Illness, Terminal
Medication
Mental Illness
Metabolic Disease

Neurological Disease
Paralysis
Renal Disease
Reproductive Problems

6. SEXUAL DYSFUNCTION RELATED TO VALUES CONFLICT

Client Responses and/or Situations Needing Assessment

WELLNESS ORIENTED

Abortion
Adolescence
Agedness
Divorce
Education, Change in
Employment, Change in
Insomnia

Life Style, Change in
Marital Status, Change in
Middle Age
Pregnancy
Relocation
Retirement
Young Adulthood

ILLNESS ORIENTED

Alcoholism
Illness, Chronic

Illness, Terminal
Substance Abuse

7. SEXUAL DYSFUNCTION RELATED TO LACK OF PRIVACY

Client Responses and/or Situations Needing Assessment

WELLNESS ORIENTED

Crowded Living Conditions
Travel

Vacations
Visitors

ILLNESS ORIENTED

Hospitalization   Illness, Chronic

8. SEXUAL DYSFUNCTION RELATED TO LACK OF SIGNIFICANT OTHER

Client Responses and/or Situations Needing Assessment

WELLNESS ORIENTED

Coping, Ineffective Family   Incarceration
Crisis, of Family   Loss, of Loved One
Death   Marital Status, Change in
Distant Family   Relocation
Divorce   Separation
Family, Single Parent

ILLNESS ORIENTED

Emotional Disorders   Illness, Terminal
Illness, Chronic   Hospitalization

9. SEXUAL DYSFUNCTION RELATED TO ALTERED BODY STRUCTURE OR FUNCTION

Client Responses and/or Situations Needing Assessments

WELLNESS ORIENTED

Anorexia/Overeating   Weight Gain
Impotence   Weight Loss
Obesity

ILLNESS ORIENTED

Amputation   Anorexia Nervosa

Body Defacement
Bulimia
Emotional Disorders
Hysterectomy
Illness, Chronic

Illness, Terminal
Mastectomy
Surgery, Facial
Tubal Ligation
Vasectomy

DIAGNOSTIC CATEGORY:
SKIN INTEGRITY, IMPAIRMENT OF:
ACTUAL

†*Definition:* A condition in which the individual has an alteration in skin integrity.

Defining Characteristics

Disruption of skin surface
Destruction of skin layers
Invasion of body structures

Nursing Diagnoses Based on Identified Etiologies

Actual Impairment of Skin Integrity Related to External (Environmental)
Actual Impairment of Skin Integrity Related to Internal (Somatic)

1. ACTUAL IMPAIRMENT OF SKIN INTEGRITY RELATED TO EXTERNAL (ENVIRONMENTAL)

A. HYPERTHERMIA OR HYPOTHERMIA

Client Responses and/or Situations Needing Assessment

280

WELLNESS ORIENTED

Cold, Excessive   Heat, Excessive
Frostbite   Sunburn

ILLNESS ORIENTED

Exposure, to Cold   Treatments, Cold
Exposure, to Heat   Treatments, Heat
Surgery, Cybernetic

B. CHEMICAL SUBSTANCE

Client Responses and/or Situations Needing Assessment

WELLNESS ORIENTED

Allergies   Poison, Plants
Medications

ILLNESS ORIENTED

Burns, Caustic   Medications

C. MECHANICAL FACTORS

Client Responses and/or Situations Needing Assessment

(*Explanation*: This diagnosis includes shearing forces, pressure, and restraints.)

WELLNESS ORIENTED

Agedness   Crutches
Casts   Diagnostic Procedures

ILLNESS ORIENTED

Alcoholism   Bedrest

Confusion
Dressings
Emotional Disorders
Level of Consciousness,
  Decreased

Mental Illness
Postoperative Period,
  Extended
Substance Abuse
Traction

D. RADIATION
Client Responses and/or Situations Needing Assessment

ILLNESS ORIENTED

Cancer
Radiation

X-rays, Excessive

E. PHYSICAL IMMOBILITY
Client Responses and/or Situations Needing Assessment

WELLNESS ORIENTED

Agedness
Allergies
Circulation, Decreases in
Depression, Moderate

Fatigue
Obesity
Stress/Distress

ILLNESS ORIENTED

Bedrest, Prolonged
Chemotherapy
Cough, Severe
Depression, Severe
Diabetes Mellitus
Diaphoresis
Fever
Fluid and Electrolyte
  Imbalance
Hospitalization, Long-Term

Illness, Chronic
Illness, Terminal
Immobility
Mental Illness, Catatonia
Metabolic Disease
Nutritional Deficiencies
Postoperative Period
Radiation Therapy
Vomiting

282 F. HUMIDITY

Potential Client Problems and/or Situations Needing Assessment

WELLNESS ORIENTED

Diarrhea

Diaphoresis

Exposure, Wet

Humidity, High

Incontinence, of Feces

Incontinence, of Urine

ILLNESS ORIENTED

†See Diagnostic Category: Bowel Elimination, Alteration in Diarrhea

†See Diagnostic Category: Bowel Elimination, Alteration in Incontinence

†See Diagnostic Category: Urinary Elimination, Alteration in Patterns

2. ACTUAL IMPAIRMENT OF SKIN INTEGRITY RELATED TO INTERNAL (SOMATIC)

A. MEDICATION

Potential Client Problems and/or Situations Needing Assessment

ILLNESS ORIENTED

Medication

B. ALTERED NUTRITIONAL STATE

Potential Client Problems and/or Situations Needing Assessment

WELLNESS ORIENTED

†See Diagnostic Category: Nutrition, Alteration in: Less Than Body Requirements

†See Diagnostic Category: Nutrition, Alteration in: More
  Than Body Requirements

ILLNESS ORIENTED

†See Diagnostic Category: Nutrition Alteration in: Less
  Than Body Requirements
†See Diagnostic Category: Nutrition Alteration in: More
  Than Body Requirements

C. ALTERED METABOLIC STATE

Client Responses and/or Situations Needing Assessment

WELLNESS ORIENTED

Adolescence	Stress/Distress
Agedness	Weight Gain
Altered Diet	Weight Loss
Anxiety	

ILLNESS ORIENTED

Diabetes Mellitus	Metabolic Disease
Endocrine Disease	

D. ALTERED CIRCULATION

Client Responses and/or Situations Needing Assessment

WELLNESS ORIENTED

Agedness	Obesity
Allergies	Pregnancy
Birth, Premature	Smoking
Circulation, Decreased	

ILLNESS ORIENTED

Bedrest	Cardiopulmonary Disease

Cardiovascular Disease	Illness, Chronic
Diabetes Mellitus	Illness, Terminal
Dialysis	Respiratory Disease

E. ALTERED SENSATION

Client Responses and/or Situations Needing Assessment

ILLNESS ORIENTED

Brain Tumor	Spinal Cord Lesion
Neurological Disease	

F. ALTERED PIGMENTATION

Client Responses and/or Situations Needing Assessment

WELLNESS ORIENTED

Nevi	Sunburn

ILLNESS ORIENTED

Cancer, Skin	Nevi
Disease Process	

G. SKELETAL PROMINENCE

Client Responses and/or Situations Needing Assessment

WELLNESS ORIENTED

Agedness	Casts
Birth, Premature	Emaciation

ILLNESS ORIENTED

Bedrest	Illness, Chronic
Cancer	Illness, Terminal
Endocrine Disease	Immobility

Level of Consciousness, Comatose
Level of Consciousness, Decreased
Metabolic Disease
Muscular Sclerosis
Musculoskeletal Disease
Neurological Disease
Neuromuscular Disease
Nutrition, T.P.N.
Nutritional Deficiencies
Nutritional Disease
Paralysis
Spinal Cord Injury
Spinal Cord Lesion

H. DEVELOPMENTAL FACTORS

Client Responses and/or Situations Needing Assessment

WELLNESS ORIENTED

Acne
Adolescence
Agedness
Birth, Premature
Obesity

I. IMMUNOLOGICAL DEFICIT

Client Responses and/or Situations Needing Assessment

ILLNESS ORIENTED

Blood Dyscrasias
Collagen Disease
Endocrine Disease
Infections
Medication, Side Effects of
Metabolic Disease
Renal Disease
Substance Abuse

J. ALTERATIONS IN TURGOR (Change in Elasticity)

Client Responses and/or Situations Needing Assessment

WELLNESS ORIENTED

Agedness
Allergies
Anorexia/Overeating
Birth, Premature

Diarrhea   Obesity
Emaciation

ILLNESS ORIENTED

Alcoholism   Hyperalimentation
Anorexia Nervosa   Malnutrition
Bulimia   Nutritional Deficiencies
Cancer   Nutritional Disease
Dehydration   Parenteral Therapy
Fluid and Electrolyte   Respiratory Disease
  Imbalance   Vomiting

K. EXCRETIONS/SECRETIONS

Client Responses and/or Situations Needing Assessment

See Diagnostic Category: Bowel Elimination, Alteration in:
  Diarrhea
See Diagnostic Category: Bowel Elimination, Alteration in:
  Incontinence
See Diagnostic Category: Urinary Elimination, Alteration
  in Patterns of

WELLNESS ORIENTED

Diaphoresis   Humidity, High
Diarrhea   Incontinence, of Feces
Exposure, Wet   Incontinence, of Urine

ILLNESS ORIENTED

Endocrine Disease   Metabolic Disease

L. PSYCHOGENIC

Client Responses and/or Situations Needing Assessment

WELLNESS ORIENTED

Allergies   Psoriasis
Anorexia/Overeating

ILLNESS ORIENTED

Anorexia Nervosa   Emotional Disorders
Bulimia   Mental Illness

M. EDEMA

Client Responses and/or Situations Needing Assessment

WELLNESS ORIENTED

Muscle Sprain   Posture, Poor
Positioning   Sunburn

ILLNESS ORIENTED

Burns   Renal Disease
Cardiopulmonary Disease   Respiratory Disease
Cardiovascular Disease   Trauma
Musculoskeletal Disease

DIAGNOSTIC CATEGORY: SKIN INTEGRITY, IMPAIRMENT OF: POTENTIAL

†*Definition:* A condition in which the individual is at risk for having an alteration in skin integrity.

Defining Characteristics

External (environmental)
    Hypothermia or hyperthermia
    Chemical substance

  Mechanical factors
    Shearing forces
    Pressure
    Restraint
  Radiation
  Physical immobilization
  Excretions and secretions
  Humidity
Internal (somatic)
  Medication
  Alterations in nutritional state (obesity, emaciation)
  Altered metabolic state
  Altered circulation
  Altered sensation
  Altered pigmentation
  Skeletal prominence
  Developmental factors
  Alterations in skin turgor (change in elasticity)
  Psychogenic
  Immunologic

Nursing Diagnoses Based on Identified Etiologies

Not applicable

DIAGNOSTIC CATEGORY: SLEEP PATTERN DISTURBANCE

Definition: Disruption of sleep time which causes individual discomfort or interferes with the individual's desired life style.

Defining Characteristics

††Verbal complaints of difficulty in falling asleep

[^††]Awakening earlier or later than desired
[^††]Interrupted sleep
[^††]Verbal complaints of not feeling well rested
  Changes in behavior and performance
    Increasing irritability
    Restlessness
    Disorientation
    Lethargy
    Listlessness
  Physical signs
    Mild, fleeting nystagmus
    Slight hand tremor
    Ptosis of eyelid
    Expressionless face
  Thick speech with mispronunciation and incorrect words
  Dark circles under eyes
  Frequent yawning
  Changes in posture
  Not feeling well rested

Nursing Diagnoses Based on Identified Etiologies

(*Explanation*: These nursing diagnoses are related to sensory alterations.)

Sleep Pattern Disturbance Related to Internal Factors
Sleep Pattern Disturbance Related to External Factors

1. SLEEP PATTERN DISTURBANCE RELATED TO INTERNAL FACTORS

A. ILLNESS

Client Responses and/or Situations Needing Assessment

ILLNESS ORIENTED

Alcoholism
Ammonia, Elevated
Brain Tumor
BUN, Elevated
Cardiovascular Disease
Cerebral Vascular Problems
CNS Depression
Congenital Abnormalities
Fluid and Electrolyte
   Imbalance

Hypoxia
Infections, Ear
Medication, Stimulants
Neurological Disease
Pain
Poison, Ingested
Substance Abuse
Surgery, Oral
Tracheostomy
Trauma

B. PSYCHOLOGICAL STRESS

Client Responses and/or Situations Needing Assessment

WELLNESS ORIENTED

Agedness
Anxiety
Childhood
Coping, Ineffective
   Individual
Crisis, of Family
Crisis, of Individual

Depression, Moderate
Fear
Knowledge Deficit
Perception, Inaccurate
Powerlessness
Stimuli, Lack of

ILLNESS ORIENTED

Alcoholism
Level of Consciousness,
   Comatose
Level of Consciousness,
   Decreased

Mental Illness
Mental Problems
Substance Abuse

2. SLEEP PATTERN DISTURBANCE RELATED TO EXTERNAL FACTORS

A. ENVIRONMENTAL CHANGES

Client Responses and/or Situations Needing Assessment

WELLNESS ORIENTED

Agedness
Crisis, of Family
Crisis, of Individual
Diagnostic Studies
Grieving
Incarceration

Infant, Incubator
Social Isolation
Tests/Treatments
Travel
Weather

ILLNESS ORIENTED

Hospitalization
Illness, Chronic
Illness, Sudden
Intensive Care Units

Isolation, Hospital
Mental Illness
Mental Illness, Paranoia
Surgery

B. SOCIAL CUES

Client Responses and/or Situations Needing Assessment

WELLNESS ORIENTED

Adolescence
Anorexia
Divorce
Economic Status, Change in
Employment, Loss of
Failure, Perceived
Financial Problems
Insomnia
Life Style, Change in

Loss, of Loved One
Loss, of Personal Items
Marital Status, Change in
Middle Age
Powerlessness
Rape Trauma
Self-Esteem, Lowered
Social Status, Change in
Young Adulthood

ILLNESS ORIENTED

Alcoholism

Anorexia Nervosa

DIAGNOSTIC CATEGORY: SOCIAL ISOLATION

Definition: Condition of aloneness experienced by the individual and perceived as imposed by others and as a negative or threatened state.

Defining Characteristics

OBJECTIVE	SUBJECTIVE
Absence of supportive significant other(s)—family, friends, group	Expresses feeling of aloneness imposed by others
Sad, dull affect	Expresses feelings of rejection
Inappropriate or immature interests and activities for developmental age or stage	Experiences feeling of difference from others
Uncommunicative, withdrawn; no eye contact	Expresses values acceptable to subculture, but unable to accept values of dominant culture
Preoccupation with own thoughts; repetitive, meaningless actions	Inadequacy or absence of significant purpose in life
Projects hostility in voice, behavior	Inability to meet expectations of others
Seeks to be alone or exists in subculture	Insecurity in public
Evidence of physical and/or mental handicap or altered state of wellness	Expresses interests inappropriate to developmental age or stage
Shows behavior unaccepted by dominant cultural group	

Nursing Diagnoses Based on Identified Etiologies

(*Explanation*: These diagnoses include factors that contribute to the absence of satisfying personal relationships.)

Social Isolation Related to Delay in Accomplishing Developmental Tasks
Social Isolation Related to Immature Interests
Social Isolation Related to Alterations in Physical Appearance
Social Isolation Related to Alterations in Mental State
Social Isolation Related to Unaccepted Social Behavior
Social Isolation Related to Unaccepted Social Values
Social Isolation Related to Altered State of Wellness
Social Isolation Related to Inadequate Personal Resources
Social Isolation Related to Inability to Engage in Satisfying Personal Relationships

1. SOCIAL ISOLATION RELATED TO DELAY IN ACCOMPLISHING DEVELOPMENTAL TASKS

Client Responses and/or Situations Needing Assessment

WELLNESS ORIENTED

Adolescence
Childhood
Crisis, of Family
Crisis, of Individual
Divorce
Economic Status, Change in
Employment, Change in
Employment, Loss of

Failure, Perceived
Financial Problems
Loss, of Personal Items
Marriage, Childless
Mental Retardation
Powerlessness
Self-Esteem, Lowered
Separation

294 Social Isolation   Support Systems, Lack of
Social Status, Change in

ILLNESS ORIENTED

Accidents   Illness, Chronic
Alcoholism   Illness, Terminal
Emotional Disorders   Mental Illness
Hospitalization   Substance Abuse
Illness, Acute

2. SOCIAL ISOLATION RELATED TO IMMATURE INTERESTS

Client Responses and/or Situations Needing Assessment

WELLNESS ORIENTED

Adolescence   Child Abuse/Neglect
Agedness   Childhood

ILLNESS ORIENTED

Alcoholism   Bulimia
Anorexia Nervosa   Substance Abuse

3. SOCIAL ISOLATION RELATED TO ALTERATIONS IN PHYSICAL APPEARANCE

Client Responses and/or Situations Needing Assessment

WELLNESS ORIENTED

Adolescence   Self-Esteem, Lowered
Agedness   Skin Changes
Anorexia/Overeating   Weight Gain
Obesity   Weight Loss

ILLNESS ORIENTED

Alcoholism
Amputation
Anorexia Nervosa
Body Defacement
Bulimia
Burns

Hysterectomy
Mastectomy
Paralysis
Skin Integrity, Impaired
Substance Abuse
Trauma, Facial

4. SOCIAL ISOLATION RELATED TO ALTERATIONS IN MENTAL STATE

Client Responses and/or Situations Needing Assessment

See Diagnostic Category: Fear

WELLNESS ORIENTED

Agedness
Anxiety
Depression, Moderate
Failure, Perceived

Fear
Powerlessness
Self-Esteem, Lowered

ILLNESS ORIENTED

Alcoholism
Anorexia Nervosa
Body Defacement
Bulimia
Depression, Severe
Emotional Problems

Mental Illness, Paranoia
Mental Illness, Suicidal
  Ideation
Mental Illness, Withdrawn
Phobias
Substance Abuse

5. SOCIAL ISOLATION RELATED TO UNACCEPTED SOCIAL BEHAVIOR

Client Responses and/or Situations Needing Assessment

WELLNESS ORIENTED

Depression, Moderate   Hyperactivity
Homosexuality   Promiscuity

ILLNESS ORIENTED

Alcoholism   Incontinence, of Urine
Incontinence, of Feces   Substance Abuse

6. SOCIAL ISOLATION RELATED TO UNACCEPTED SOCIAL VALUES

Client Responses and/or Situations Needing Assessment

WELLNESS ORIENTED

Abortion   Insomnia
Adolescence   Life Style, Change in
Anorexia/Overeating   Loss, of Loved One
Coping, Ineffective Family   Loss, of Personal Items
Coping, Ineffective Individual Marital Status, Change in
Culture/Values   Powerlessness
Divorce   Rape Trauma
Economic Status, Change in   Self-Esteem, Lowered
Failure, Perceived   Social Status, Change in
Financial Problems

7. SOCIAL ISOLATION RELATED TO ALTERED STATE OF WELLNESS

Client Responses and/or Situations Needing Assessment

WELLNESS ORIENTED

Wellness, Change in Level of

ILLNESS ORIENTED

Cancer
Diagnosis, New
Illness, Chronic

Illness, Sudden
Illness, Terminal

8. SOCIAL ISOLATION RELATED TO INADEQUATE PERSONAL RESOURCES

Client Responses and/or Situations Needing Assessment

WELLNESS ORIENTED

Crisis, of Family
Crisis, of Individual
Divorce
Economic Status, Change in
Family Separation
Financial Problems
Knowledge Deficit

Loss, of Loved One
Marital Status, Change in
Relocation
Resources, Lack of
Retirement
Separation
Support Systems, Lack of

9. SOCIAL ISOLATION RELATED TO INABILITY TO ENGAGE IN SATISFYING PERSONAL RELATIONSHIPS

Client Responses and/or Situations Needing Assessment

WELLNESS ORIENTED

Adolescence
Agedness
Blindness
Childhood
Deafness
Depression, Moderate

Failure, Perceived
Infancy
Marital Status, Change in
Middle Age
Powerlessness

Self-Esteem, Lowered

Separation

Separation, from Loved One

Tests/Treatments

Young Adulthood

ILLNESS ORIENTED

Depression, Severe

Hospitalization

Illness, Chronic

Illness, Terminal

Mental Illness

DIAGNOSTIC CATEGORY: SPIRITUAL DISTRESS (Distress of the Human Spirit)

Definition: Distress of the human spirit is a disruption in the life principle that pervades a person's entire being and that integrates and transcends one's biologic and psychosocial nature.

Defining Characteristics

††Expresses concern with meaning of life and death and/or belief systems

Anger toward God (as defined by the person)

Questions meaning of suffering

Verbalizes inner conflict about beliefs

Verbalizes concern about relationship with deity

Questions meaning for own existence

Unable to choose or chooses not to participate in usual religious practices

Seeks spiritual assistance

Questions moral and ethical implications of therapeutic regimen

Displacement of anger toward religious representatives

Description of nightmares or sleep disturbances

Alteration in behavior or mood evidenced by anger,

crying, withdrawal, preoccupation, anxiety, hostility, apathy.
Regards illness as punishment
Does not experience that God is forgiving
Is unable to accept self
Engages in self-blame
Denies responsibilities for problems
Description of somatic complaints

Nursing Diagnoses Based on Identified Etiologies

Spiritual Distress Related to Separation from Religious and Cultural Ties

Spiritual Distress Related to Challenged Belief and Value System

1. SPIRITUAL DISTRESS RELATED TO SEPARATION FROM RELIGIOUS AND CULTURAL TIES

Client Responses and/or Situations Needing Assessment

WELLNESS ORIENTED

Adolescence
Agedness
Coping, Ineffective Family
Coping, Ineffective Individual
Crisis, of Family
Crisis, of Individual
Depression, Moderate
Divorce
Family Separation
Marital Status, Change in
Relocation
Separation
Stress/Distress
Support Systems, Lack of
Young Adulthood

ILLNESS ORIENTED

Bedrest

Body Defacement

300

Hospitalization
Hospitalization, Prolonged
Illness, Sudden
Illness, Terminal
Intensive Care Units

Isolation
Nutrition, Effect of Diet
 Restrictions on
Pain
Paralysis

2. SPIRITUAL DISTRESS RELATED TO CHALLENGED BELIEF AND VALUE SYSTEM

(*Explanation*: This diagnosis is the result of moral or ethical implications of therapy or result of intense suffering.)

Client Responses and/or Situations Needing Assessment

WELLNESS ORIENTED

Abortion
Anorexia/Overeating
Crisis, of Family
Crisis, of Individual
Death
Loss, of Loved One

Loss, of Personal Items
Rape Trauma
Sleep Disturbance
Social Isolation
Weight Loss

ILLNESS ORIENTED

Illness, Chronic
Illness, Terminal
Medications
Pain
Surgery, Impending

Tests/Treatments, Invasive
Tests/Treatments, Painful
Transfusions
Transplant Surgery,
 Impending

DIAGNOSTIC CATEGORY: THOUGHT PROCESSES, ALTERATION IN

†*Definition:* A condition in which the individual is unable to use the cognitive process to maintain activities of daily living.

Defining Characteristics

Inaccurate interpretation of environment
Cognitive dissonance
Distractibility
Memory deficit or problems
Egocentricity
Hyper/hypovigilance
Decreased ability to grasp ideas
Impaired ability to make decisions
Impaired ability to problem solve
Impaired ability to reason
Impaired ability to abstract or conceptualize
Impaired ability to calculate
Altered attention span—distractibility
Commands; obsessions
Inability to follow
Disorientation to time, place, person, circumstances, and events
Changes in remote, recent, immediate memory
Delusions
Ideas of reference
Hallucinations
Confabulation
Inappropriate social behavior
Altered sleep patterns
Inappropriate affect
Inappropriate/nonreality-based thinking

Nursing Diagnoses Based on Identified Etiologies

Alteration in Thought Processes Related to Physiologic Changes

Alteration in Thought Processes Related to Psychologic Conflicts

Alteration in Thought Processes Related to Loss of Memory

Alteration in Thought Processes Related to Impaired Judgement

Alteration in Thought Processes Related to Sleep Deprivation

1. ALTERATION IN THOUGHT PROCESSES RELATED TO PHYSIOLOGIC CHANGES

Client Responses and/or Situations Needing Assessment

WELLNESS ORIENTED

Agedness   Mental Retardation

ILLNESS ORIENTED

Alcoholism   Level of Consciousness,
Brain Tumor   Lowered
Cardiovascular Disease   Neurological Disease
Cerebral Vascular Problems   Substance Abuse
Congenital Abnormalities

2. ALTERATION IN THOUGHT PROCESSES RELATED TO PSYCHOLOGIC CONFLICTS

Client Responses and/or Situations Needing Assessment

WELLNESS ORIENTED

Adolescence	Failure, Perceived
Anxiety	Fear
Crisis, of Family	Powerlessness
Crisis, of Individual	Rape Trauma
Depression, Moderate	Stress/Distress

ILLNESS ORIENTED

Depression, Severe	Mental Illness,
Emotional Disorders	Schizophrenia
Mental Illness	Mental Illness, Suicidal
Mental Illness, Paranoia	Ideation

3. ALTERATION IN THOUGHT PROCESSES RELATED TO LOSS OF MEMORY

Client Responses and/or Situations Needing Assessment

WELLNESS ORIENTED

Agedness	Sleep Deprivation
Amnesia	Social Isolation
Depression, Moderate	Stress/Distress
Fear	

ILLNESS ORIENTED

Cardiovascular Disease	Isolation
Cerebral Vascular Problems	Neurological Disease

4. ALTERATION IN THOUGHT PROCESSES RELATED TO IMPAIRED JUDGEMENT

Client Responses and/or Situations Needing Assessment

WELLNESS ORIENTED

Agedness	Infancy
Anxiety	Mental Retardation
Childhood	Stress/Distress
Fear	

ILLNESS ORIENTED

Alcoholism	Hallucinations
Cardiovascular Disease	Mental Illness
Cerebral Vascular Problems	Neurological Disease
Delusions	Substance Abuse
Emotional Disorders	

5. ALTERATION IN THOUGHT PROCESSES RELATED TO SLEEP DEPRIVATION

Client Responses and/or Situations Needing Assessment

WELLNESS/ILLNESS ORIENTED

See Diagnostic Category: Sleep Pattern Disturbance

DIAGNOSTIC CATEGORY: TISSUE PERFUSION, ALTERATION IN: CEREBRAL, CARDIOPULMONARY, RENAL, GASTROINTESTINAL, PERIPHERAL

†*Definition:* A condition in which the individual experiences a decrease in blood supply to a body part.

Defining Characteristics

Characteristic	Chances defining characteristic will be present given diagnosis	Chances defining characteristic not explained by any other diagnosis
Skin temperature: cold extremities	High	Low
Skin color		
Dependent, blue or purple	Moderate	Low
††Pale on elevation, and color does not return on lowering leg	High	High
††Diminished arterial pulsations	High	High
Skin quality: shining	High	Low
Lack of lanugo	High	Moderate
Round scars covered with atrophied skin		
Gangrene	Low	High
Slow-growing, dry, thick, brittle nails	High	Moderate
Claudication	Moderate	High
Blood pressure changes in extremities		
Bruits	Moderate	Moderate
Slow healing of lesions	High	Low

††Critical defining characteristic.

Comment: Further work and development are required for three subcomponents of this diagnosis, specifically cerebral, renal, and gastrointestinal.

306 **Nursing Diagnoses Based on Identified Etiologies**

(*Explanation*: These diagnoses may be specified to include cerebral, cardiopulmonary, renal, gastrointestinal, and peripheral.)

Alteration in Tissue Perfusion: (Specify) Related to Interruption of Flow, Arterial

Alteration in Tissue Perfusion: (Specify) Related to Interruption of Flow, Venous

Alteration in Tissue Perfusion: (Specify) Related to Exchange Problems

Alteration in Tissue Perfusion: (Specify) Related to Hypervolemia

Alteration in Tissue Perfusion: (Specify) Related to Hypovolemia

1. ALTERATION IN TISSUE PERFUSION: (SPECIFY) RELATED TO INTERRUPTION OF FLOW, ARTERIAL

Client Responses and/or Situations Needing Assessment

WELLNESS ORIENTED

Agedness	Obesity
Anorexia/Overeating	

ILLNESS ORIENTED

Cancer	Embolus
Cardiopulmonary Disease	Endocrine Disease
Cardiovascular Disease	Infection
Congenital Abnormalities	Metabolic Disease
Congestive Heart Failure	Nutritional Disease

Renal Disease   Trauma
Respiratory Disease   Tumor
Tests/Treatments, Invasive

2. ALTERATION IN TISSUE PERFUSION: (SPECIFY) RELATED TO INTERRUPTION OF FLOW, VENOUS

Client Responses and/or Situations Needing Assessment

WELLNESS ORIENTED

Agedness   Obesity
Anorexia/Overeating

ILLNESS ORIENTED

Cancer   Metabolic Disease
Cardiopulmonary Disease   Nutritional Disease
Cardiovascular Disease   Renal Disease
Congenital Abnormalities   Respiratory Disease
Congestive Heart Failure   Tests/Treatments, Invasive
Embolus   Trauma
Endocrine Disease   Tumor
Infection

3. ALTERATION IN TISSUE PERFUSION: (SPECIFY) RELATED TO EXCHANGE PROBLEMS

Potential Client Problems and/or Situations Needing Assessment

WELLNESS ORIENTED

Agedness   Altitude, High
Allergies   Aspiration

308

Birth, Premature   Newborn
Cough, Chronic

ILLNESS ORIENTED

Blood Dyscrasias   Infection, Lung
Cancer   Peripheral Vascular Disease
Cardiopulmonary Disease   Renal Disease
Cardiovascular Disease   Respiratory Disease
Congenital Abnormalities   Respiratory Distress
Embolus   Syndrome
Fluid and Electrolyte   Surgery
   Imbalance

4. ALTERATION IN TISSUE PERFUSION: (SPECIFY) RELATED TO HYPERVOLEMIA

Client Responses and/or Situations Needing Assessment

ILLNESS ORIENTED

Alcoholism   Hypothermia
Cardiopulmonary Disease   Malnutrition
Cardiovascular Disease   Metabolic Disease
Congestive Heart Failure   Parenteral Therapy
Endocrine Disease   Renal Disease
Fluid Volume, Excess   Water Intoxication
Hyperalimentation

5. ALTERATION IN TISSUE PERFUSION: (SPECIFY) RELATED TO HYPOVOLEMIA

Client Responses and/or Situations Needing Assessment

ILLNESS ORIENTED

Anorexia Nervosa
Burns
Dehydration
Dialysis
Diaphoresis
Diarrhea

Endocrine Disease
Hemorrhage
Hyperthermia
Metabolic Disease
Vomiting

DIAGNOSTIC CATEGORY: URINARY ELIMINATION, ALTERATION IN PATTERNS OF

†*Definition:* A condition in which the individual experiences a change in urinary function.

Defining Characteristics

Dysuria
Frequency
Hesitancy
Incontinence

Nocturia
Retention
Urgency

Nursing Diagnoses Based on Identified Etiologies

Alteration in Patterns of Urinary Elimination Related to Sensory Motor Impairment

Alteration in Patterns of Urinary Elimination Related to Neuromuscular Impairment

Alteration in Patterns of Urinary Elimination Related to Mechanical Trauma

1. ALTERATION IN PATTERNS OF URINARY ELIMINATION RELATED TO SENSORY MOTOR IMPAIRMENT

310 **Client Responses and/or Situations Needing Assessment**

WELLNESS ORIENTED

Agedness	Enuresis
Childhood	Fear
Drugs	

ILLNESS ORIENTED

Anesthesia	Neurological Disease
Anorexia Nervosa	Nutritional Disease
Cerebral Vascular Problems	Paralysis
Congenital Abnormalities	Renal Disease
Infection	Spinal Cord Injury
Malnutrition	Spinal Cord Lesion
Mental Illness, Catatonia	

2. ALTERATION IN PATTERNS OF URINARY ELIMINATION RELATED TO NEUROMUSCULAR IMPAIRMENT

Client Responses and/or Situations Needing Assessment

WELLNESS ORIENTED

Agedness	Enuresis
Childhood	Pregnancy

ILLNESS ORIENTED

Alcoholism	Level of Consciousness, Decreased
Anesthesia	
Cerebral Vascular Problems	Neurological Disease
Congenital Abnormalities	Neuromuscular Disease
Level of Consciousness, Comatose	Organic Brain Syndrome
	Paralysis

Renal Disease	Substance Abuse
Spinal Cord Injury	Surgery, Renal
Spinal Cord Lesion	Surgery, Urinary Tract

3. ALTERATION IN PATTERNS OF URINARY ELIMINATION RELATED TO MECHANICAL TRAUMA

Client Responses and/or Situations Needing Assessment

ILLNESS ORIENTED

Congenital Abnormalities	Paralysis
Musculoskeletal Disease	Trauma, Musculoskeletal

DIAGNOSTIC CATEGORY: VIOLENCE, POTENTIAL FOR: SELF-DIRECTED OR DIRECTED AT OTHERS

[†]*Definition:* A condition in which the individual exhibits behaviors indicative of an impending violent action.

Defining Characteristics

Body language: clenched fists, facial expressions, rigid posture, tautness indicating intense effort to control

Hostile threatening verbalizations; boasting of prior abuse to others

Increased motor activity, pacing, excitement, irritability, agitation

Overt and aggressive acts; goal-directed destruction of objects in environment

Possession of destructive means: gun, knife, weapon

Rage

Self-destructive behavior and/or active, aggressive suicidal acts

Substance abuse or withdrawal
Suspicion of others, paranoid ideation, delusions, hallucinations
Increasing anxiety level
Fear of self or others
Inability to verbalize feelings
Repetition of verbalizations; continued complaints, requests, and demands
Anger
Provocative behavior; argumentative, dissatisfied, overreactive, hypersensitive
Vulnerable self-esteem
Depression (specifically active, aggressive, suicidal acts)

Nursing Diagnoses Based on Identified Etiologies

Explanation: These nursing diagnoses may be specified to include violence that is self-directed or directed at others.

Potential For Violence: (Specify)

1. POTENTIAL FOR VIOLENCE: (SPECIFY)

Client Responses and/or Situations Needing Assessment

ᵃILLNESS ORIENTED

Antisocial Character
Battered Women
Catatonic Excitement
Child Abuse
Manic Excitement
Organic Brain Syndrome

Panic States
Rage Reactions
Suicidal Behavior
Temporal Lobe Epilepsy
Toxic Reactions to Medicatio

ᵃThese client responses and situations were identified as etiologies according to NANDA.